María del Pilar Díaz Martínez

Physical Therapy Assessment

María del Pilar Díaz Martínez

Physical Therapy Assessment

Strategies and tools for evaluation

ScienciaScripts

Cover image: www.ingimage.com

This book is a translation from the original published under ISBN 978-613-9-43469-5.

Publisher:
Sciencia Scripts
is a trademark of
Dodo Books Indian Ocean Ltd. and OmniScriptum S.R.L publishing group

120 High Road, East Finchley, London, N2 9ED, United Kingdom
Str. Armeneasca 28/1, office 1, Chisinau MD-2012, Republic of Moldova, Europe
Printed at: see last page
ISBN: 978-620-8-19160-3

Index

1. Historical foundations of physiotherapy

The history of physical therapy dates back to ancient times, where physical agents such as water, heat and massage were used in combination with magical or religious rituals to cure illnesses. In ancient Greece, Hippocrates promoted self-healing of the body by natural means and mentioned the therapeutic use of water and massage. During the Middle Ages, there was a decline in the use of these methods due to religious prohibitions, but in the Renaissance the classical approach was resumed and massage therapy was recommended for various ailments (1).

In the sixteenth and seventeenth centuries, works were published highlighting the importance of physical exercise and massage therapy for health. In the 18th century, authors such as Antonio Pérez Escobar and Joseph Clement Tissot advocated the incorporation of physical exercise in medical treatment. In the 19th century, with the advent of evolutionism and positivism, there were great advances in medicine and science, although physical agents still did not occupy a prominent place compared to surgery and pharmacology. During this period, important contributions were made in the field of physiotherapy, such as the development of physical education by Pehr Henrik Ling, the introduction of mechanotherapy by Zander, and the studies of electrostimulation by Duchenne De Boulogne. These advances laid the foundation for the evolution of physiotherapy as a therapeutic discipline in the following centuries (1).

During the 20th century, physiotherapy underwent a significant development that marked its consolidation as a health care discipline. In the early years of the century, the publication of "Gilbert and Carnot's Library of Therapeutics" introduced the term "physiotherapy" and classified physical agents for the first time. Prominent practitioners such as Frenkel, Klapp and Lovett, among others, made important contributions to the treatment of various conditions, from cerebellar disorders to scoliosis and muscular imbalances. In 1933, Guthrie-Smith developed the apparatus that would bear his name, which laid the foundation for what is known today as poleotherapy. In 1946, Delorme and Watkins designed a systematic muscle strengthening method called "progressive resistance exercises", contributing to the evolution in the treatment of muscle strength. Françoise Mézières initiated the study of muscle chains in 1949, laying the foundations of modern techniques such as global postural reeducation and the muscle chain technique. Herman Kabat developed the proprioceptive neuromuscular facilitation method in the 1940s, focusing on muscular potentiation and proprioception. In 1958, the World Health Organization (WHO) defined physiotherapy as "the art and science of treatment by means of therapeutic exercise, heat, cold, water, massage and electricity". In 1967, the World Confederation for Physical Therapy (WCPT) described it as "the art and science of physical treatment," focusing on the use of physical agents to cure, prevent, recover and readapt patients. The Bobath couple introduced a treatment technique for infantile cerebral palsy, which was later extended to the treatment of adults with hemiplegia. In 1967, Hislop and Perrine developed the concept of "isokinetic work", which revolutionized treatment by means of resistance proportional to the muscular force exerted. Václav Vojta published in 1974 a system of early diagnosis and treatment based on postural reactivity, especially relevant in the pediatric field (2).

Among the events of physiotherapy in Spain, March 2, 1969 stands out, with a meeting in Madrid that marked the beginning of the foundation of the Spanish Association of Physiotherapists (AEF). Subsequently, on June 12, 1969, in Barcelona, the Constituent Assembly was held where the first National Board of Directors, led by José Llopis Diez, was approved and confirmed. In 1970, the AEF underwent significant changes with the election of a new board of directors during an assembly in Alicante, headed by Mr. Roberto González Fernández. That same year, the AEF joined the European Confederation of Physiotherapists, strengthening its position at the international level. The AEF was dedicated to promoting the elevation of physiotherapy studies to university level, working closely with the Ministry of Education to establish the University Schools of Physiotherapy in line with international standards. During the following years, the AEF worked on the elaboration of a new curriculum for physiotherapy, leading a national commission in charge of this project. In 1972, the association submitted to the Ministry of Education a project for the restructuring of physiotherapy studies, which eventually led to the promulgation of a Royal Decree in 1980, establishing the basis for the creation of the University Schools of Physiotherapy. In parallel, the AEF consolidated its international presence by being recognized as a full member of the World Confederation of Physiotherapists in 1974. In addition, it continued to promote the profession nationally, organizing events and conferences, and launching the magazine "Fisioterapia" in 1979. In June of that year, a general assembly was held in which a new national board of directors was elected, led by Mr. Roberto Núñez Pérez, marking the beginning of a new era for physiotherapy in Spain (3).

Physiotherapy experienced significant progress in Spain from the 1980s onwards, with important milestones that contributed to its development and recognition as a university degree and health profession. In 1980, physiotherapy was established as a university degree in Spain, but it was in 1987, with the University Reform Law, when it received an important boost. During these years, the Spanish Association of Physiotherapists (AEF) made active efforts in favor of the growth of the profession. In 1985, the AEF adapted its Statutes to the new territorial organization, and in 1989, the Official University Degree in Physiotherapy was officially established. The integration of the physiotherapist in the Primary Care team, promoted by the AEF, marked an important milestone in 1989, followed by a more detailed regulation in 1991. In addition, in 1989, the "Specific Area of Knowledge of Physiotherapy" was consolidated, allowing physiotherapists access to academic positions (3).

In 1990, the First International Congress of Sports Physiotherapy in Spain was held in Valladolid. However, the most significant milestone was the foundation of the first professional association of physiotherapists in the country: the Association of Physiotherapists of Catalonia, supported and financed by the Spanish Association of Physiotherapists (AEF). This step marked the beginning of the creation of professional associations in all the autonomous communities, making the members of the AEF the first collegiate members. In 1998, the General Council of Associations of Physiotherapists of Spain defined physiotherapy as "the science and art of physical treatment", focused on the use of physical means to cure, prevent disease and promote health. In 1999, the World Confederation for Physical Therapy (WCPT) updated the definition of physical therapy, emphasizing that it is a service provided by physical therapists, which includes assessment, diagnosis, planning, intervention and evaluation, and that complete and functional movement is fundamental to health. In 2001, the AEF commemorated the 50th anniversary of the WCPT and signed an agreement to organize its XIV World Congress. Scientific publications were also promoted. In 2002, Mrs. Antonia Gómez Conesa became the first physiotherapist to obtain a University Chair. These events marked significant milestones in the consolidation and recognition of physiotherapy as a vital health profession in Spain (4).

Throughout the following years, significant milestones have been reached in the development and promotion of physiotherapy in Spain. In 2003, the XIV WCPT Congress was held in Barcelona and the Permanent Board of the AEF was renewed. In 2004, the White Paper on the Degree in Physiotherapy was published and the Official College of Physiotherapists of La Rioja was created. Student movements in 2005 advocated for quality training, while in 2006 the Technical Sheet for Undergraduate Studies in Physiotherapy was published and the foundations were laid for the Iberoamerican Association of Physiotherapy and Kinesiology. In 2007, the 50th anniversary of physiotherapy in Spain was celebrated and the conditions of the Study Plans for the Degree in Physiotherapy were approved. In 2008, the Permanent Board of the AEF was renewed and the sponsorship of the PEDro database was approved. Since 2012, the Revista Iberoamericana de Fisioterapia y Kinesiología merged with the journal Fisioterapia. In 2012, Madrid hosted the XIV National Congress of Physiotherapy, standing out for its innovation and active participation. In November of that year, during the X Anniversary of the Professional Association of Physiotherapists of Extremadura, Ms. Antonia Gómez Conesa was elected as president of the Permanent Board. In December 2014, new regulations were approved to improve the functioning of the AEF and it was decided that Antonia Gómez would continue as editor of the journal after her presidency. During this decade, the AEF promoted the creation of specialized affiliate associations, such as the Spanish Association of Physiotherapists in Mental Health and others. She collaborated with the ER-WCPT in the creation of the European Physiotherapy Guidelines for Parkinson's Disease. From 2010 to 2016, Sonia Souto represented the AEF as Second Vice Chairman of the ER-WCPT. The AEF actively participated with the Ministry of Health in various strategies and projects, such as the IMA Project (Intelligent Motion Analysis) and the Commitment to Quality of Scientific Societies Project. In 2016, the journal Fisioterapia obtained the seal of Quality of

Scientific Journals. In addition, the AEF organized two international events in Madrid in collaboration with WCPT (1).

2. Physiotherapist's performance

2.1. Functions of the physical therapist.

According to Royal Decree 1001/2002 of September 27, 2002, physiotherapy is a health profession that focuses on the prevention, evaluation, diagnosis and treatment of musculoskeletal and neurological disorders, as well as on promoting the well-being and quality of life of the individual. It is based on the use of manual techniques, therapeutic exercises, physical agents and patient education to restore physical function and improve mobility, strength and flexibility. Physiotherapy addresses both acute and chronic dysfunctions, working in collaboration with other health professionals to achieve the best results for the patient (5).

The function is what defines the exercise of a profession. According to the statute of the General Council of Colleges of Physiotherapists, Chapter I of the basic principles of the practice of Physiotherapy, in Article 1 Of Physiotherapy we find that Physiotherapy is the study and art of physical treatment, that is, the set of methods, actions and techniques that, through the application of physical means, heal and prevent disease, promote health, recover, train, rehabilitate and readapt people affected by psychophysical dysfunctions or those who want to maintain an adequate level of health. The practice of Physiotherapy also includes the performance by the physiotherapist, alone or in a multidisciplinary team, of electrical and manual tests aimed at determining the degree of affectation of innervation and muscle strength, tests to determine functional capacities, range of joint movement and measures of vital capacity, all focused on determining the physiotherapeutic evaluation and diagnosis, as a preliminary step to any act of physiotherapy, as well as the use of diagnostic aids to monitor the evolution of users. The ultimate goal of physiotherapy is to promote, maintain, restore and increase the level of health of citizens in order to improve the quality of life of the person and facilitate their full social reintegration (5).

In Article 2 Of Physiotherapists, we find the responsibilities of the physiotherapist, whether in terms of care, teaching, research or management, derive directly from the primary role of physiotherapy in society. These responsibilities are carried out in accordance with the fundamental ethical principles that govern all professional practice. This implies a profound respect for the dignity of the person, the protection of their human rights, as well as a marked responsibility, honesty and sincerity in all interactions with users. Within these responsibilities is the task of establishing and applying a wide range of physical means with therapeutic effects in treatments for users of various medical and surgical specialties. These physical means include, among others, the application of electricity, heat, cold, massage, water, air, movement, light and specialized therapeutic exercises. Such interventions are applied in areas such as cardiopulmonary, orthopedics, neurological injuries, pre- and postpartum maternity, among others. It also includes the performance of specific manual procedures and treatments, alternative or complementary, within the scope of physiotherapy (5).

These responsibilities are performed in a variety of settings, ranging from health institutions to educational centers, sports facilities, physical therapy offices, rehabilitation centers and gyms, among others. Once physical therapists comply with the requirements established by the applicable legislation, they acquire full rights and faculties to practice their profession, regardless of the modality or legal title under which they provide their services. It is important to emphasize that the free practice of the profession of physical therapist takes place in a context of free competition and is subject to specific regulations, particularly with regard to the offer of services and the determination of remuneration, in accordance with current legislation on antitrust and unfair competition (5).

2.2. Levels of performance.

The first step in systematizing the action of physical therapists involves understanding that health systems are complex structures involving organized relationships between the population and institutions. In the face of health challenges and needs, an organized social response by health institutions is crucial. Health systems are organized around basic functions and organizational arrangements for health promotion, protection, cure and rehabilitation.

The proposed model emphasizes that the action of physical therapists in health systems involves a dynamic relationship between the population, with its demands and needs, and the institutions that provide health services. Physiotherapists have a crucial role in primary health care (PHC), secondary care, tertiary care, health surveillance and health management.

- Regarding primary health care, its importance is recognized in order to improve access, increase resolution and expand the comprehensiveness of care. However, there are challenges in the clear definition of the role of the physical therapist at this level of care. It is proposed that, in PHC, the physiotherapist should articulate clinical, prevention and health promotion activities. This implies a clinical and individualized care, which strengthens the contact with users and increases resolution. The model suggests the creation of physiotherapy units in PHC, organized territorially and linked to family health teams. The distribution of the workload among different types of activities contributes to define the purposes and responsibilities of physiotherapeutic work at this level. In addition, the idea of direct access to physiotherapy is proposed, allowing patients to go directly to the physiotherapist without the need for medical referral. This strengthens professional autonomy and reduces organizational barriers in health services (6).
- In tertiary care, Physiotherapy is performed in the hospital and in specialized centers that are linked to the hospital, aimed at the sick individual suffering from medical and surgical diseases that generally require more advanced methods for their treatment than those used at the primary level (6).
- In terms of health surveillance, the physical therapist has an important role in protecting the health of the population, participating in risk control measures and monitoring of diseases, injuries and disabilities. This extends to all spheres of health surveillance, such as sanitary, epidemiological, worker and environmental surveillance (6).

Finally, the model highlights the role of the physiotherapist in the management of health systems, including the coordination of multiprofessional teams, the management of health units and participation in the formulation of public policies. Expanding the scope of action of physical therapy in health systems leads to a better level of health and greater independence and functionality of the population (6).

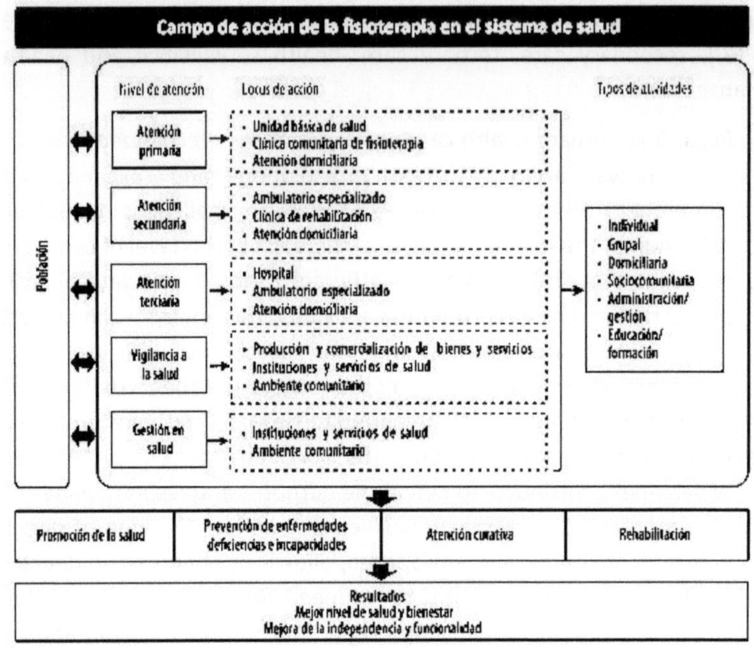

Figure 1. Conceptual framework of the physical therapist's field of action in health systems (6).

3. Methodology of intervention in physiotherapy (MIF)

Physical therapy intervention methodology is a systematic and organized method of administering individualized physical therapy care that focuses on identifying and treating the unique responses of individuals or groups to actual or potential health disturbances. This method goes by several names, Heerkens calls it the "Physical Therapy Process", while Rebollo calls it the "Physical Therapy Intervention Method (PIM)". This methodology consists of five stages (1):

- 1st Stage. Assessment: Collection and analysis of information to determine the patient's health status and to describe the patient's capabilities and problems (actual or potential). Includes referrals, physical therapy history, physical examination and registration.
- 2nd Stage. Data analysis: Identification of real or potential problems that can be solved by the physiotherapist or referred to other professionals. The physiotherapy diagnosis is established.
- 3rd Stage. Formulation of the physical therapy program: Establishment of problems, objectives and interventions.
- 4th Stage. Implementation of the program: Execution of the physical therapy plan, applying the planned methods and techniques, collecting information on the patient's response and recording the patient's data and responses.
- 5th Stage. Evaluation: Verification of the effectiveness of the physiotherapy program and decision on the need to make changes. If the objectives have not been achieved, the method is reviewed to correct errors and achieve the formulated objectives.

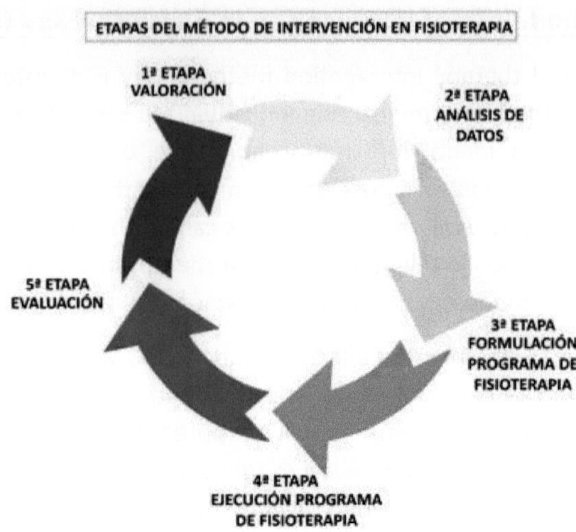

Figure 2. Representation of the physiotherapy intervention method (1).

4. Aspects of physical therapy assessment

Assessment is the first stage of the MIF, where all relevant data about the patient are collected and recorded in order to obtain as accurate an understanding of the patient's health condition as possible. The principles that compose it are (1):

4.1. Anamnesis.

The anamnesis is a colloquial process in which the patient is interviewed (direct anamnesis) or his/her relatives or companions if necessary. This process can present difficulties. It is crucial to adapt the language and terminology to the patient so that he/she can understand the information. A cordial and pleasant atmosphere should be created during the interview. It is important to allow the patient to express him/herself freely. Use terms that the patient can understand. Questions should be direct, specific and understandable. It is essential to know how to listen to the patient and give him/her the necessary time to express him/herself. The anamnesis is the first step in the interaction with the patient, during which information about the patient's health status, personal history and health-related conditions is collected in an orderly and detailed manner, with the aim of making an accurate physiotherapeutic diagnosis (7).

The patient is the main source of data. This is the fundamental starting point for gathering information. The patient, being the party directly affected by the health condition, can provide accurate data about himself, including symptoms, previous medical history, current medications, and other details relevant to diagnosis and treatment. Their subjective perception of their health status and experiences are vital to a full understanding of the clinical situation. The patient's family can be a valuable source of information, especially in situations where the individual is unable to provide accurate data, such as in cases of loss of consciousness, dementia, or similar situations. Family members can provide information about the patient's medical history, recent changes in health status, medications, allergies, and other relevant aspects. In addition, the family can offer additional insights into the patient's behavior and health, which may be useful to complement the information provided by the patient himself and to obtain a more complete picture of the clinical situation (1).

4.2. Medical history.

The medical record is a document whose main purpose is to organize information related to the patient's health in order to facilitate patient care. Therefore, when an individual needs health services, the health personnel must prepare and keep his or her medical history updated over time. The definition of medical records can be approached from various perspectives, such as grammatical, legal and health care. From the latter point of view, the document records all the interventions and activities carried out by healthcare personnel related to the patient's health, with the aim of improving healthcare from the moment of birth to the end of life. This medical record must be configured in such a way as to be an effective tool in the interprofessional care process. According to article 3 of Law 41/2002, which regulates patient autonomy and the rights and obligations regarding clinical information and documentation, the medical record is defined as the set of documents containing information on the clinical situation and evolution of a patient during his or her care (7).

Thus, the clinical history in physiotherapy fulfills several functions, among which the following stand out (7):

- Assistance: with the purpose of providing the patient with the most appropriate medical care.
- Educational: detailing and explaining the therapeutic and exploratory decisions taken, demonstrating the correct approach in the treatment and management of clinical cases.
- Clinical research: developing a set of categories to classify and group medical records involving a specific pathology, clinical case or intervention.
- Epidemiological research: grouping cases in clinical research using appropriate population denominators.
- Clinical management and medical resource planning: in the organization and evaluation of available resources for future investment planning.
- Legal and juridical aspects: recording all care received by the patient in order to establish documentary evidence.

- Care quality control: quantifying and evaluating the complete process of medical care to the patient, with an evaluation of the scientific and technical aspects.

The clinical record in the specialty of physical therapy is a legal instrument and an essential component in patient care. This record should include a series of key elements for each patient in order to ensure comprehensive and quality care. The following are the components that should be present in the physical therapy clinical record (7):

The patient's history includes several fundamental elements. First, the patient's personal data should be collected, such as name, age, sex, address, telephone number and any other relevant identifying information. Next, the reason for admission or consultation should be specified, i.e., the reason why the patient has come to the physical therapy office, whether it is a medical recommendation, an injury, a specific pain or any other cause. It is also essential to include a detailed description of the patient's present medical condition, including symptoms, duration of symptoms and any other relevant details. In addition, it is important to record family history, which includes information about relevant diseases or medical conditions in the patient's family that may have an impact on the patient's current health. On the other hand, personal history includes the patient's personal medical history, including previous illnesses, treatments received, allergies, among others. It is crucial to include relevant information from the patient's birth, including childhood and adolescence, as this data may influence the patient's current condition. Finally, the patient's habits should be described, such as smoking, alcohol consumption, physical activity, diet, among others.

The patient's medical history should also be detailed. This includes the surgical history, which is a record of all surgeries the patient has had, with dates, reasons and results. It should also include the medical history, which is a list of all the diseases and medical conditions the patient has had throughout his or her life. The work history is another key piece, as it provides information about the patient's work, including possible occupational hazards that may affect his or her health. It is essential to list all current medication the patient is taking, with dosage and frequency. In addition, a systematic history of the present medical condition, which is a detailed and chronological description of the evolution of the patient's current medical condition, should be included.

The physical evaluation is another essential component of the clinical record. This includes a clinical evaluation of the skin, an evaluation of the subcutaneous tissue and an evaluation of the skin structures for potential problems. An evaluation of the head and neck should also be performed, as well as palpation of the lymph nodes to identify possible swelling or abnormalities. Evaluation of the neuro-musculoskeletal system is crucial to identify any problems in these systems. In addition, the distribution of pain in the patient's body should be recorded and analyzed. It is important to include a physical examination of the respiratory system and an evaluation of the circulatory system to detect possible problems in these systems. Assessment of functionality and independence in activities of daily living is a key aspect of physical therapy. This includes a summary and clinical conclusions based on the evaluation performed. The therapy used and treatments applied to the patient during the physical therapy process should also be detailed. A provisional syndromic diagnosis should be established based on the symptoms and the initial evaluation, as well as complementary diagnostic methods used to complement the initial diagnosis. The definitive diagnosis is established after the complete evaluation and complementary diagnostic methods. It is essential to establish short, medium and long term objectives for the patient's recovery and improvement, with specific goals in different time frames. The physiotherapeutic intervention plan should be detailed and personalized. In addition, a prognosis, which is a prediction of the likely course of the patient's condition and recovery, should be provided. Follow-up is crucial and should include recording of follow-up sessions and ongoing assessment of the patient's progress. Finally, you should record the patient's discharge upon completion of treatment and provide a follow-up report detailing the patient's progress after discharge, including recommendations for the maintenance of the patient's health.

This scheme allows for a comprehensive and organized collection of all relevant patient information, ensuring that physiotherapy treatment is effective and personalized.

In addition to the patient, the patient's family and the medical history, there are other relevant sources of information in the medical field, such as (1):

- Nursing records: These records contain crucial data on the patient's daily care, including medication administration, vital signs, procedures performed and any significant changes in the patient's condition. They are an important source for tracking the patient's progress during his or her stay in the health care facility.
- Physical therapy report: This report details the patient's physical evaluation, clinical findings, physical therapy treatment plan and progress made during therapy. It includes information on therapeutic exercises, mobilization techniques, preventive and rehabilitative measures, as well as recommendations for ongoing patient management.
- Occupational therapy reports: These reports provide information on the patient's functional ability in activities of daily living, such as self-care, mobility, and participation in social and work activities. They also include therapeutic goals, intervention strategies and progress during occupational therapy.
- Psychological reports and tests: These reports provide a detailed assessment of the patient's mental and emotional state. They include diagnoses, psychological test results, observations on behavior and emotional state, as well as recommendations for therapeutic intervention.

These additional sources of information are essential for a comprehensive patient assessment and for effective, personalized treatment planning.

4.3. Clinical interview.

Data collection in physical therapy takes place at the initial interview and is obtained from various sources such as the user, family members, caregivers, previous physical therapy records, health history and diagnostic tests. During this first consultation, it is crucial to gain the patient's trust by complying with certain basic rules of behavior: do not rush, avoid interruptions, be observant and respect the patient's privacy. For this, it is necessary to have an adequate space. It is also important to obtain information on the patient's beliefs and expectations regarding the healthcare system, medication use, behavioral patterns, work, socio-family and economic impact. All this information should be recorded in the physiotherapy record, which is an integral part of the patient's health history, thus ensuring that his or her passage through the unit and how his or her problem has been addressed within the healthcare system is documented. During the interview, it is essential to use clear communication, with short sentences, using drawings if necessary, and to verify the patient's degree of understanding and opinion on the subject (8).

For an effective interview, it is recommended to follow the five-step rule (8):

- Listening: Allow the patient to express him/herself freely to encourage openness in future sessions. Avoid forming a rigid idea from the first interview.
- Assess: Use intelligent palpation and observation of the patient's motor behavior to identify motor and painful problems. Although there may be differences from what the patient has reported, do not contradict the patient's perception of discomfort.
- Interrogate: To deepen the initial answers without suggesting answers to the patient.
- Observe: Listen to the description of symptoms and observe the patient's behavioral signs to ensure consistency between narrative and observation.
- Understanding: Clearly expressing that the patient's difficulties have been understood and that they are not indifferent to the therapist.

To facilitate the physical therapist-patient relationship, some ideas are suggested (8):

- Use the patient's own name.
- Introduce yourself and show interest in the patient's problem, without minimizing the symptoms expressed by the patient.
- Explain the purpose of the questions to provide better care.
- Maintain good eye contact and give full attention to the patient.
- Devote the necessary time, since haste shows disinterest.
- Plan the interview in advance to better control the time available.

4.4. Physical examination of the patient

In the physical examination the objective is to identify the structures or factors responsible for the patient's symptoms. Physical tests are performed to find signs that confirm or rule out the hypothesis that the structures identified in the subjective examination are actually the source of the symptoms. Two key aspects are assumed during the physical examination:

- Symptom Reproduction: If symptoms are reproduced when evaluating a structure, the symptoms are considered to originate from that structure. However, it is difficult to establish an accurate structural diagnosis as the tests affect multiple tissues, both proximal and distal. For example, knee flexion affects not only the joint, but also the capsule, ligaments, muscles, surrounding nerve tissue, and the joints, muscles and nerves of the proximal hip and spine, as well as the distal ankle.
- Anomaly Detection: If an anomaly is detected in a structure that could theoretically refer symptoms to the affected area, that structure is considered to be the suspected source of the symptoms. This anomaly is described as a "comparable" referral sign (Maitland, 1991).

In the physical examination, data are collected through observable and measurable information. For this, various resources are used, such as visual, manual, instrumental and functional:

4.4.1. Visual resources:

It is crucial that the physiotherapist obtains information from what he/she observes in the patient such as general condition, posture, gait, etc. The diversity and multiplicity of possible observations do not allow an exhaustive list to be presented. However, it is necessary to remember that only those observations that can contribute to therapeutic action should be recorded, and that the recording should be done with all possible guarantees.

Observation in the context of neuromusculoskeletal assessment is the comprehensive and systematic process by which the therapist visually examines the patient to identify any abnormalities, dysfunction or signs of pathology. This assessment is performed at different times and positions to obtain a complete understanding of the patient's condition. Observation is of great importance as we can identify pathology, detect visual signs of various conditions, such as inflammation, muscle atrophy, and deformities. It helps to identify elements that may be aggravating the patient's condition, such as poor posture, incorrect movement patterns and inappropriate use of aids. It serves as a guide for testing and treatment; the information obtained through observation directs the therapist as to what tests to perform and what therapeutic approaches may be most effective. Observation can be both informal and formal (9).

- Informal Observation: The therapist should observe the patient in both dynamic and static situations. This observation includes the quality of the patient's movement, postural characteristics and facial expression. The goal is to assess the quality of the patient's movement and postural characteristics in a natural and unstructured manner. It is carried out during the initial conversation and general observation of the patient in everyday situations, such as entering the room, sitting or standing up. It allows the therapist to pick up on spontaneous behaviors of the patient that may not be evident during a more structured assessment. Details of Informal Observation (9):
  - Movement Quality: Evaluate how the patient moves, observing fluidity, coordination and any restrictions or abnormalities in their movements.
  - Postural Characteristics: Examine the patient's alignment and posture while standing and sitting. This may reveal muscle misalignments or strains that are not readily seen in a formal evaluation.
  - Facial Expression: Observe the patient's facial expressions, as they may provide clues to pain or discomfort that may not be verbalized.
  - Use of Aids: Check whether the patient is using aids such as neck braces, canes or corsets, and whether they are being used correctly. This includes observing for visible bandages, which may indicate possible disease behavior.
  - Supplemental Information: Informal observation can provide as much valuable information as formal assessment. This is because patients may not adopt their usual posture during a structured assessment, but do so in a more relaxed and less conscious environment.
  - Behavioral Identification: The manner in which the patient uses orthopedic aids may give clues about his or her health status and attitude toward his or her condition. For example, a visible bandage may suggest a disease behavior or pain management strategy.

- Formal observation: Formal observation in physical therapy involves a structured and systematic evaluation of the patient, following specific protocols and tools. This observation is performed in a methodical manner and is designed to objectively document the physical and functional status of the patient. For this purpose we can use (9):
  - Standard Assessments: Use standardized tools and questionnaires to measure pain intensity, location and characteristics (e.g., visual analog pain scale).
  - Functional Testing: Perform specific physical tests to assess mobility, strength, flexibility and other functional aspects of the patient.
  - Detailed Documentation: Accurate and detailed recording of findings during the assessment for proper follow-up and treatment planning.

4.4.2. Manual resources:

- Palpation:

Palpation is a fundamental technique in the evaluation that consists of tactile compression with the palmar aspects of the fingers or fingertips. Through this technique, the physical therapist can assess a variety of characteristics in the patient's body that are crucial for the diagnosis and follow-up of various health conditions (10, 11). Philip Greenman, in his splendid analysis Principles of Manual Medicine (Greenman, 1989), summarizes the five objectives of palpation. The practitioner or therapist must be able to (12):

- Detect abnormal tissue texture.
- Examine the symmetry in the position of the structures, both tactilely and visually.
- Detect and assess variations in the arc and quality of movement during the stroke, as well as the quality of the end of the arc of any movement.
- Sense the position in space of oneself and the person being palpated.
- Detect and evaluate changes in the palpated data, whether they have improved or worsened over time.

Some characteristics that should be assessed when performing a skin fold are (10, 11):

- Flexibility, elasticity, thickness, consistency or trophic condition: Some of the aspects that are evaluated by palpation is the elevation or depression of the skin, detecting any areas that are abnormally raised or sunken compared to the surrounding tissue, which may indicate the presence of inflammation, masses, scars or lesions.
- Temperature: Palpation allows the skin temperature to be assessed, identifying areas that are warmer or colder than normal, which may be a sign of infection, inflammation, circulation problems or changes in blood flow.
- Arterial and venous pulses: Palpation is crucial for checking pulses in different parts of the body. By palpating superficial arteries such as those in the wrists, neck or ankles, the strength, rhythm and regularity of the pulse can be assessed, providing vital information about cardiovascular function and blood flow.
- Diaphoresis (sweating)
- Swelling, edema and inflammation: Another important application is the assessment of the contours and size of organs and tumors. By palpation of the abdomen, the size and shape of internal organs such as the liver and spleen can be determined, as well as detecting the presence of masses or tumors that may require further evaluation.
- Hypersensitivity: Hypersensitivity is another characteristic that is examined through palpation, identifying areas where the patient feels increased pain or unusual sensitivity to touch, which may be indicative of inflammation, injury, infection or other pathological conditions.
- Lymph nodes: Evaluation of the lymph nodes is another important application of palpation, as they may become enlarged or swollen in response to infection, autoimmune disease or cancer. Through palpation, the physical therapist can detect these changes and assess the consistency, mobility and tenderness of the affected nodes.
- Contralateral comparison and adjacent areas: In the examination of each body system, palpation and tissue mobilization require attention to the region involved, constant comparisons with the other side, and exploration in different anatomical planes in an

orderly and sequential manner. This technique provides accurate information or indications of possible deficiencies that should be confirmed or ruled out in other examinations.

- Joint crepitus: A crunching sensation or sound felt when moving a joint, which can be a sign of joint diseases such as arthritis. This procedure requires the physical therapist to have a broad knowledge of anatomy in order to identify alterations, asymmetries and deviations in different types of tissues, including bone, joint, capsule-ligament, muscle, aponeurotic, tendon, nerve, skin, adipose tissue, blood vessels, masses, inflammation, edema and loss of tissue continuity.
- Skin mobility with respect to underlying tissues: Tissue mobilization provides valuable information on the location, extent and severity of some structural and functional deficiencies of the involved body segments. In other words, the purpose of palpation and tissue mobilization is to locate the origin of pain (if present) and to identify structural and functional deficiencies that may compromise the function of one or more body systems, as well as the patient's emotional condition, which affects human body movement and, therefore, the normal development of daily activities and social participation. The tactile exploration carried out by the physical therapist requires comparing the findings of palpation in loading postures with those of rest. Resting postures require the patient to be comfortable and relaxed, while some abnormalities are only perceived during activity, so it is necessary to complement palpation with other examination procedures.

There are several types of palpation according to their depth (10, 11):

- By performing superficial palpation, we can process information about skin changes, temperature changes, superficial muscle tension, provoked pain and edema.
- On deep palpation, if we increase the pressure on palpation, we obtain information about provoked pain, tissue mobility, edema, deep muscle tension, fibrosis and interosseous changes.

Types of palpation the technique used (10, 11):

- Flat palpation: Performed with the end of the finger, it facilitates the mobility of the subcutaneous cellular tissue, useful in superficial musculature and abdomen.
- Pincer palpation: Useful in bulky belly muscles.
- Deep palpation: Used when it is not possible to perform a pincer or flat palpation, to produce sensitivity in the muscle.

Practice is essential to develop palpation and gain expertise. Thinking hands" refers to the mind's attention to the structures palpated, identifying variations in these structures. Modulating the pressure applied ensures that accurate information is obtained without causing pain to the patient.

It is important to consider the type of structure being explored (10, 11):

- Artery: Its pulsatile rhythm is perceived.
- Vein: When pressed at a point, it fills up below the pressure point.
- Tendon: It is closely related to the muscle.
- Ligament: It is palpable depending on the position of the joint.

Preliminary premises (10, 11):

- The area to be palpated should be bare.
- Adopt a relaxed position.
- The arms should be supported to avoid deviations in palpation.
- The first contact should be slow and gentle.
- Repeat the palpation several times to obtain consistent results.

Palpation is a simple, practical and information-rich tool. As the physical therapist gains experience, this technique becomes more useful and important in the evaluation process. Palpation also allows differentiating the structures involved by the specific location of the pain, being important to determine the characteristics of the hypersensitivity found. Investigating the particularities of the pain helps the physical therapist to classify its cause as neurogenic, musculoskeletal or vascular. Neurogenic pain is characterized by being widespread, sharp, imprecise and following the involved nerve pathway, and may be accompanied by sensory, trophic and reflex deficits. Musculoskeletal pain, if of bony origin, is easy to localize, deep and described by patients as "drilling", increasing with digital pressure, forced postures, specific movements and, sometimes, with thermal changes. Vascular pain is widespread, permanent, referred, and is associated with pulse weakness, thermal and skin coloration changes. Identifying areas of anesthesia, allodynia, hypoesthesia, hyperesthesia or hypersensitivity to tactile exploration also helps to identify functional deficits of sensory origin. Following the distribution of segmental cutaneous innervation or the distribution map by dermatomes allows the exact location of the deficiency, although overlaps and differences between individuals should be taken into account (10, 11).

- Percussion:

Percussion has been used for both manual and diagnostic treatment for many years. Albert Abrams, in his 1910 work "Spondylotherapy", was one of the first to study this subject in depth. In his foreword, Abrams emphasized the crucial role of mechanical vibration in therapy, noting that its application is effective and practical when handled correctly. Abrams described his percussion technique using a piece of rubber or linoleum as the recipient of the blow and a large rubber head to transmit the force. He also mentioned the use of knuckles or fingers in the absence of these instruments. The linoleum strip was placed over the spinous process, applying a series of rapid and vigorous blows, which, although uncomfortable for the patient, did not cause other negative effects. Later, in 1939, Dr. A. C. Johnson discussed the use of hand or mechanical instruments to apply effective vibrations when done quickly enough. Although the text does not elaborate on the therapeutic use of percussion, it highlights its diagnostic value. Percussion has historically been used to define the position and status of organs, with variations in its use in Eastern and Western medicine. A wide range of sounds can be interpreted, as detailed by Sir Robert Hutchinson in 1897. He described how percussion can identify the location of organs and variations in their resonance. For example, Hutchinson discussed thoracic percussion, describing both qualitatively and quantitatively the sounds (hyperresonance, dullness, timpanic timbre, etc.). These variations have diagnostic and prognostic value (12).

Regarding the method used to perform percussion, Hutchinson recommended using the middle finger of the left hand as a pleximeter, applied firmly over the tissues to be percussed, with no air between the finger and the skin, and tapped with the middle finger of the right hand. The method involves tapping from the wrist, lifting the finger after the tap to allow vibration, similar to a piano mechanism. For firmer percussions, multiple fingers can be used, but generally one finger is sufficient. Three key rules according to Hutchinson (12):

- Percuss from resonant (hollow) to less resonant (solid) areas.
- Keep the pleximeter finger parallel to the edge of the organ and perpendicular to the percussion line.
- Ensure close contact between the pleximeter finger and the tissues.

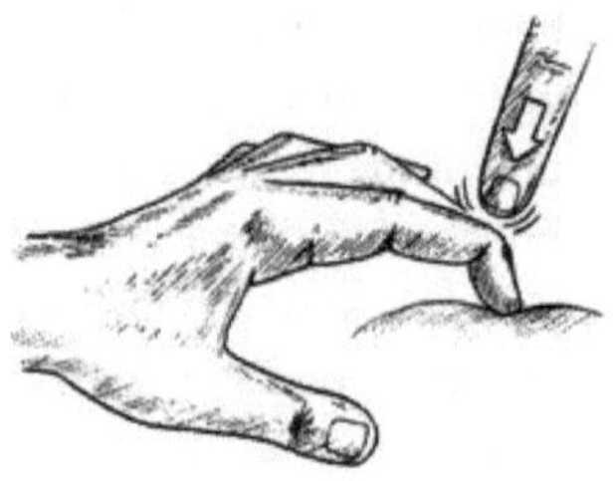

Figure 3. Position of the final phalanx kept as vertical as possible with respect to the surface examined, as indicated by Abrams (12).

On abdominal percussion, Hutchinson noted that the sound depends on the depth of the airspace and the tension of the organ wall. The presence of gas in the peritoneal cavity can eliminate the normal dullness of the liver or spleen. If there is abnormal dullness, it should be verified if it is maintained in all positions or changes with the movement of the patient, important to distinguish between gas, ascites, or tumors (12).

4.4.3. Instrumental resources:

Instruments and scales are used to perform analytical assessments to examine the different organic structures separately, considering their behavior in a normal state. These means mainly assess three parameters: flexibility, strength and coordination and balance (1):

- Flexibility: The goniometer and the tape measure are used for its evaluation. Goniometers are used to quantify joint angulation or amplitude. The tape measure measures perimeters, contours and lengths.

- Strength: Determines the extent and amplitude of muscle weakness. Originally devised by Lovett, they have been improved with numerical systems by Lowman and percentage records by Henry O. and Florence P. Kendall. Currently, the Lovett scale with Lowman gradation is used, ranging from 0 (inactive muscle) to 5 (normal muscle). This evaluation is based on three elements: palpation of the contraction, the action of gravity and the application of an external force. Other scales to evaluate muscle weakness are the Daniels, Williams and Worthingham scale. This scale assesses muscles in relation to the force of gravity, which is taken as the standard resistance. Another instrument used to assess muscle strength is the dynamometer. Isokinetic methods can also be used, which provide objective and reproducible information on muscle strength. These exercises, devised by James Perrine, allow the maximum possible force and angular movement to be exerted at a constant speed.
- Coordination and balance:
  - Simple Methods: These include activities such as walking in a straight line, standing on one foot or touching your nose with your eyes closed.
  - Complex Methods: The MOVE (Mobility Opportunities Via Education) method improves mobility through comprehensive education. Although designed for children, it is also applicable to adults. This method uses 16 categories of key motor skills, from the simplest to the most complex, assessing 74 individual skills. Examples of skills include turning while upright, which involves keeping the hips and knees straight while rotating the body, with or without additional support. This method allows for an in-depth assessment of the skills needed to lead an autonomous life, also providing guidelines for their attainment.

4.4.4. Functional resources:

Functional assessments make it possible to analyze the interrelationship between the various structures of the organism, placing the person in a context of autonomy. In addition, they examine the person's motor behavior in relation to activities of daily living in his or her environment. Functional assessments aim to provide a comprehensive view of the body's functioning in everyday activities, allowing a more holistic and patient-centered approach to treatment planning and rehabilitation strategies (1):

- Greater objectivity in the measurement of functions.
- Systematization of the functional exploration.
- Detection of disabilities in early stages.
- Transmission of information and follow-up of therapeutic plans.

Both instrumental and functional means can be used, as long as they are validated and show high reliability. Validity refers to the ability of the instrument or scale to reflect what it claims to measure, and reliability refers to the ability of an instrument or scale to give the same score, in the absence of changes, when performed by more than one evaluator. The following are the degrees into which they can be classified (1):

- Classification by degree of reliability:
  - Grade 3: Total Reliability
    - Characteristics: Also called validated, these tests show a statistically proven absence of variability in the results.
    - Use: The measurements obtained can be used without risk by different teams in different countries.
    - Examples: Cobb angle or Katz daily independence index.
  - Grade 2: Reproducibility and Acceptability
    - Features: Simplicity in their operation ensures that they can be used correctly by a large number of professionals. There is general acceptance of the procedure in the interpretation and evaluation of the result.
    - Examples: Manual muscle function test, visual analog pain scale, electrocardiograms.
  - Grade 1: Viability
    - Characteristics: Reliability is affected by different standards depending on the countries and equipment using them, which prevents uniform standardization of results.
    - Use: The results can only be compared with the average range depending on the instrument used.
    - Examples: Isokinetic devices.
  - Grade 0: Imprecision
    - Characteristics: Differences between teams in the same country make it impossible to establish inter-institutional comparisons.

- Examples: Different schools of training and evaluation.

These reliability levels help determine the usefulness and accuracy of the assessment tests in various clinical and research applications.

5. Pain assessment

Pain is the main symptom that leads a patient to consult a healthcare professional. It is defined as an unpleasant sensory and emotional sensation associated with an actual or potential injury. Because pain is a subjective experience and varies between individuals, it is difficult to quantify. For this purpose, a pain assessment is performed, which will cover the following points (13):

- Communication with the Patient: It is crucial for the healthcare professional to ask the patient about his or her pain using clear language and concise questions, allowing time to respond.
- Key Questions:
  - Home: Why? What do you attribute it to? What do you think it is due to?
  - Evolution: How long have you had this discomfort? Is this the first time something like this has happened to you? Has the discomfort improved or worsened since it started? Has it changed over time? Have you consulted a physician about it?
  - Location and Intensity: Where do you notice the pain? Is it diffuse or specific? Does it radiate to another part of the body? Is it severe? On a scale of 1 to 10, how much would you give it? What relieves or increases it? Can you sleep well? Does the pain wake you up at night?
  - Time and Evolution: Do you remember how it started? Since when? Did it begin abruptly or gradually? Is it continuous or intermittent? Have you had this type of pain before? Is it frequent?
  - Quality: How would you describe the pain - is it stabbing, dull, burning, oppressive?
  - Types of Pain:
    - For Physiology:
      - Nociceptive pain: Results from somatic or visceral damage. Examples: activation of nociceptors in skin, bone, soft tissues.
      - Neuropathic pain: Result of injury or disease of the nervous system. Characterized by allodynia. Examples: trigeminal neuralgia, phantom limb pain.
    - By Location:
      - Localized: Direct relation with the stimulus, responds to anti-inflammatory drugs.
      - Irradiated: Extends along a nerve.

- Referred: Perceived in a region other than that of the origin of the pain.
- By Evolution Time:
  - Acute: Immediate result of activation of the nociceptive system due to tissue damage.
  - Chronic: Persistent, does not act as an alarm signal and may be associated with psychological symptoms.
- Qualities of Pain
  - Sharp: Pleural pain.
  - Taladrante: Periodontitis.
  - Oppressive: Angina pectoris.
  - Electric shock: Trigeminal neuralgia.
  - Burning: Herpes zoster.
  - Mild but continuous: Cancer.
  - Heaviness: Headaches due to hypertension.
  - Colic: intestinal or biliary colic.
  - Punctures: Tabes dorsal.
  - Heartbeat: Pulpitis.

5.1. Scales and questionnaires for pain assessment.

- Unidimensional Scales for Measuring Pain Intensity (14):

  - Visual Analog Scale (VAS): The Visual Analog Scale (VAS) measures pain intensity by means of a 10-centimeter horizontal line. The left end indicates no pain and the right end indicates maximum pain. The patient is asked to mark a point on the line according to his or her pain, and this mark is measured in centimeters or millimeters. The intensity is classified as mild up to 4 cm, moderate between 5 and 7 cm, and severe if greater than 7 cm.

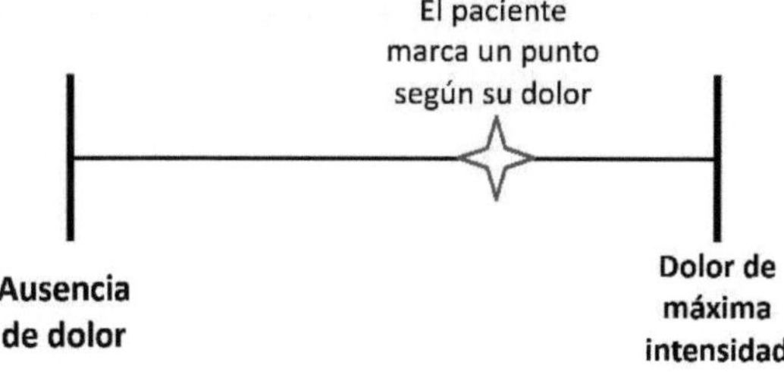

Figure 4. Visual Analog Scale (14).

- Verbal Numeric Scale (EN): The patient selects the number that best evaluates the intensity of his or her symptom. It is the simplest and most commonly used scale. The EN is a numbered scale from 0 (no pain) to 10 (maximum pain intensity).

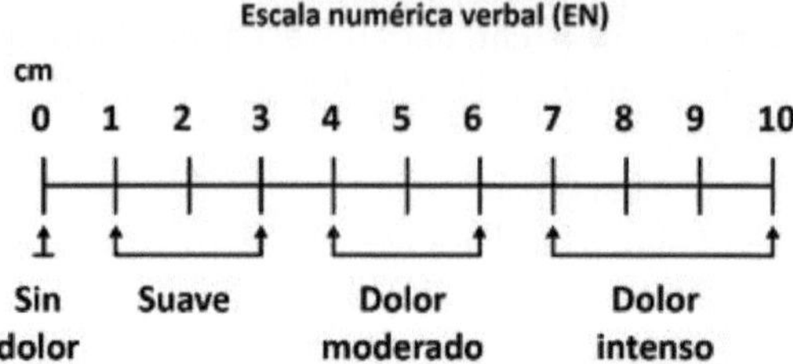

Figure 5. Verbal numerical scale (14).

- Verbal Categorical Scale (VC): The VC is used when the patient cannot quantify symptoms with other scales. It expresses the intensity of symptoms in categories, which is simpler. An association is established between categories and a numerical equivalent.

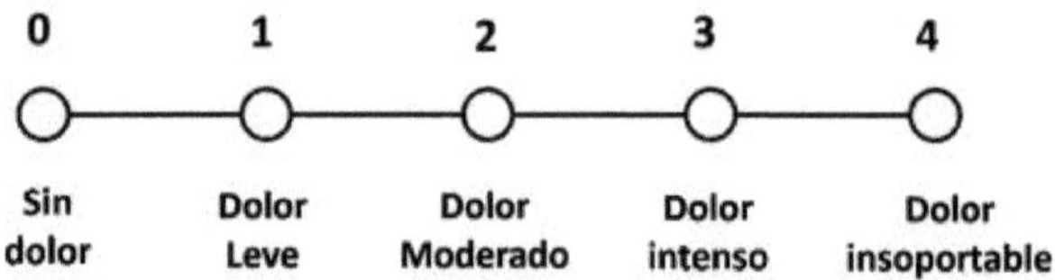

Figure 6. Verbal categorical scale (14).

- Facial Pain Scale: The Wong and Baker Facial Pain Scale, also known as the facial pain scale, is used mainly in children. It presents a series of faces with expressions ranging from joy to crying, each associated with a number from 0 (no pain) to 6 (maximum pain). The patient selects the face that best represents the intensity of his or her pain at that moment.

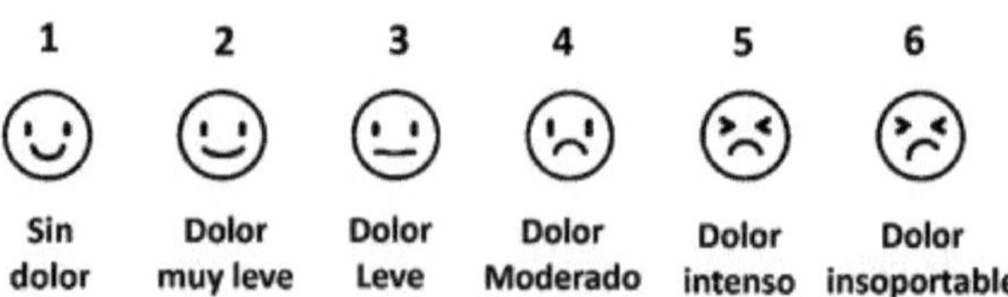

Figure 7. Facial Pain Scale (14).

Meticulously analyzing the information provided by the patient about his or her pain is essential to guide the diagnosis and plan the appropriate treatment, also considering the psychosocial aspects that may influence his or her pain experience (13).

- Multidimensional scales to measure pain:

Multidimensional scales for measuring pain are tools that allow different aspects of pain to be assessed in a comprehensive manner. Some of the most commonly used ones are presented here (15).

MULTIDIMENSIONAL PAIN SCALES	
McGill Pain Questionnaire (MPQ)	It is a widely used tool that examines the sensory and affective dimensions of pain. Patients are presented with a list of adjectives grouped into 20 subclasses, and are asked to select one adjective from each subclass that best describes their pain experience. Each adjective is associated with a specific score. This questionnaire is useful for discerning between different types of pain and has been adapted to Spanish.
The Spanish Pain Questionnaire (CDE)	It is aimed at the general population experiencing acute or chronic pain. It is self-administered and addresses various dimensions of pain, such as sensory, affective and evaluative.
The Chronic Pain Coping Questionnaire (CAD)	It is a tool that assesses how people cope with chronic pain. It consists of 31 items distributed in 6 subscales and is aimed at individuals who have experienced pain for more than 6 months.
The DN4 Questionnaire	It is a diagnostic tool for neuropathic pain consisting of seven items related to symptoms and three to clinical examination. A total score of 4/10 or higher suggests the presence of neuropathic pain. This questionnaire has been validated in Spanish and other languages.
West Haven-Yale Multidimension	It is a comprehensive tool consisting of 52 items grouped into 12 scales. It assesses several areas,

al Pain Inventory (WHYMPI)	including pain intensity, interference with the patient's daily life, perceived support and negative mood states.
The Lattinen Test	It is a tool used in Pain Units to evaluate different aspects of the patient's condition. It is easy to use and has been recently validated.
The Brief Pain Inventory (Brief Pain Inventory)	It was originally developed to assess oncologic pain. It is used in both clinical and research settings to assess the intensity and impact of pain and the effects of analgesic treatment. There are long and short versions, both validated in Spanish.
The LANSS Pain Scale and The Neuropathic Pain Questionnaire (NPQ)	They are specific tools to distinguish between neuropathic and non-neuropathic pain.
Pain DETECT	It is self-administered and also helps in this differentiation.

Table 1. Multidimensional scales to measure pain (15).

The following is a detailed observation sheet that allows us to better understand the pain experienced by the patient. This tool will help us assess the intensity, duration and characteristics of the pain, as well as identify possible triggers and relieving factors, providing a solid basis for effective diagnosis and treatment.

Hoja de observaciones para registrar las características del dolor

Fecha: Nombre: Edad:

Uso para el evaluador

Origen del dolor

Mapa corporal:

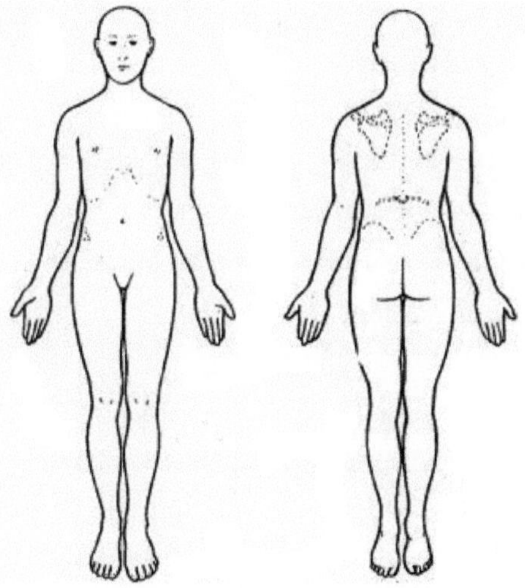

Respiratorio Neurológico Cardiaco

Osteoarticular Vascular Muscular

Otro

Evaluación del dolor

El paciente siente dolor:

Localizado Irradiado Referido

Tiempo de evolución: Agudo Crónico

Cualidades del dolor:

Punzante ☐ Taladrante ☐ Opresivo ☐ Descarga eléctirca ☐

Quemante ☐ Leve pero continuo ☐ Pesadez ☐

Colico ☐ Pinchazos ☐ Latidos ☐

Uso para el paciente

Medicamento

Analgésico: Dosificación: Hora de toma:

Tiempo que lleva administrándose:

Evaluación del dolor

¿Hace cuanto presenta dolor?:

El dolor ha:

Desaparecido ☐ Disminuido ☐ Aumentado ☐ Se mantiene igual ☐

¿El dolor ha cambiado de localización?:

¿Dónde dolía anteriormente y donde se localiza actualmente?

¿Cuá es la intensidad del dolor?.

Escala numérica verbal (EN)

0 1 2 3 4 5 6 7 8 9 10

1	2	3	4	5	6
Sin dolor	Dolor muy leve	Dolor Leve	Dolor Moderado	Dolor intenso	Dolor insoportable

¿Normalmente a qué hora comienza y termina el dolor?:

¿Qué está haciendo cuando comienza el dolor?:

¿Cómo es du dolor durante el día?:

Aumenta Disminuye ☐ Continuo ☐ Intermitente ☐ Pasajero ☐

¿Qué hace para reducir el dolor?:

Usualmente, ¿logra minimizar su dolor?:

Nunca ☐ Pocas veces ☐ Ocasionalmente ☐ Casi siempre ☐ Siempre ☐

¿Considera que el dolor va a desaparecer por completo? Explique por qué:

Qué expectativas tiene con el tratamiento fisioterapéutico:

Table 2. Observation sheet for recording pain characteristics.

Table 2. Observation sheet for recording pain characteristics.

6. Diagnosis in physiotherapy

Sahrmann, in 1988, defines physiotherapeutic diagnosis as "the term designating the essential dysfunctions that are the object of the physiotherapist's treatment. The physiotherapist identifies the dysfunctions on the basis of the history of the disease, signs, symptoms, examinations and tests that he himself performs or requests". According to Heerkens, physiotherapeutic diagnosis is "a physiotherapist's professional opinion of a patient's health status, considering the underlying pathological process and based on baseline information, history data, additional physical and medical examination data, and psychosocial data." The Standing Committee of the Union for Physiotherapy in Europe (1996) defines physiotherapeutic diagnosis as "the diagnosis established by the physiotherapist that will provide him with the indications on which to base his intervention program and its modalities of application" (16).

Physiotherapeutic diagnosis should not compete with medical diagnosis. The function of diagnosis is to make sense of a set of signs and symptoms. The physician collects abstract parameters, usually translated into figures, focusing on biological disorders and making a diagnosis that describes the patient's problems, some of which are not the purview of physical therapy. The physiotherapist investigates visible and concrete parameters of functional activity that can usually be measured (16).

6.1. Structure of the physiotherapeutic diagnosis

Any diagnosis must follow a specific structure. The elements that make it up are the following (17):

- Problems: It is defined as the whole response of the person or group to a change in their health status or situation.
- Causes: They indicate the root of the problem. They are the central axis of the physiotherapy program from which the physiotherapist will orient his action plan.
- Manifestations: These are the symptoms and signs that can be observed and assessed.
- Symptoms: Subjective manifestations of the problem expressed verbally or non-verbally, through behaviors such as anguish, apathy, sadness.

- Signs: Objective and measurable manifestations of the presence of a problem, such as limitation of joint range, muscle atrophy, etc.

The elaboration of the physiotherapeutic diagnosis follows this sequence (17):

- Collect a set of elementary signs by palpation and physical examination.
- Select a reflection nucleus, the pathognomonic element.
- Mentally establish a list of possible causes through an exhaustive interview with the patient.
- Filter the list of causes.
- Select the possible diagnosis.
- Select the necessary objectives and techniques.

6.2. Quality applied to physiotherapeutic diagnosis

Quality research is based on three important points (16):

- Objectivity: It is recommended to describe signs and symptoms accurately.
- Homogeneity: In similar cases, the therapeutic strategy will be similar, modified only on the basis of objective characteristics, if possible measured, that distinguish one patient from another. Physical therapy procedures should be analyzed, and practical training has been shown to be more important than medical training in minimizing interobserver variability.
- Reliability: Different professionals with the same measuring device on the same patient and at the same stage of evolution should obtain similar figures. If the difference is excessive, it is essential to establish standards and compare results.

6.3. Diagnostic tools

The diagnostic tools in physiotherapy are divided into three categories. In the first category we find the objectives are the goals towards which the treatment is directed. They represent the expected results that the physical therapist and the patient hope to achieve at the end of the therapeutic process. In the second category are the criteria are the reference points that allow the inclusion or exclusion of a class of patients. These criteria state or judge the patient's situation and should be considered as instruments of precision that allow the hypotheses formulated from the diagnosis to be verified. The arrangement of the criteria advises a logical organization of the treatment, thus facilitating a clear and efficient structure to address the patient's needs. In the third category, indicators are individualized elements that together may constitute a criterion. An indicator refers to a single criterion, providing a specific measure or signal that is used to assess the patient's condition. However, a criterion can encompass several indicators, integrating multiple aspects to provide a more complete and detailed view of the patient's health status. This integration allows the physical therapist to accurately monitor and adjust treatment as needed (17).

6.4. Problems and action plan

In Physiotherapy, once the pathology is known through diagnosis, the physiotherapist can evaluate the patient's disabilities, identify the problem and establish a plan of action. To plan the treatment, after the assessment and evaluation, the physiotherapist draws up a list of phenomena that need explanation, i.e. the problems, defines goals to be achieved, called objectives, and sets a deadline for their attainment. The proposed method for planning encompasses several functions. First, health problems must be identified and prioritized. Then, programs are devised and implemented to respond to these problems. Finally, the impact on health is evaluated. The characteristics of all planning include having a prospective character, which means that there is a causal relationship between the action taken and the results obtained. In addition, the process is continuous and dynamic, which means that it is constantly changing and adapting as the treatment is developed and the patient's evolution is observed (16).

7. Functioning, disability and health

7.1. International Classification of Impairments, Disabilities and Handicaps (ICIDH).

The International Classification of Impairments, Disabilities and Handicaps (ICIDH) was published in 1980 by WHO to categorize the consequences of diseases and their impact on an individual's life. This classification was intended to provide a conceptual framework for information related to the long-term consequences of diseases, injuries and other disorders. The ICIDH introduced the concepts of (18):

- Impairment: "Any loss or abnormality of a psychological, physiological or anatomical structure or function". There is a localizable and exploratory clinical manifestation, accessible by physical examination.
- Disability: "Any restriction or absence (due to an impairment) of the ability to perform an activity in the manner or within the range considered normal for a human being".
- Handicap: "A disadvantageous situation for an individual, resulting from an impairment or disability, which limits or prevents the performance of a role that is normal for him/her (depending on his/her age, sex and social and cultural factors)".

This classification was used to assess the condition of patients in rehabilitation centers, convalescent homes and nursing homes, facilitating communication between different types of care agents and the coordination of the various types of care.

- In health centers, ICIDH helped (18):
  - Determine the number and characteristics of personnel required.
  - Check the types of sick leave.
  - Analyze the modalities of utilization of health care services.
  - To provide a scientific basis with effective statistical tools and indicators to better understand the population with disabilities.
  - Determine the needs of people with disabilities and handicaps, identify disabling situations in the social and physical environment.
  - Formulate policy decisions to improve daily life, including modifications to the physical and social environment.

7.2. International Classification of Disability and Health Functioning-CIF.

ICIDH was revised and replaced by ICIDH-2 at the 54th World Health Assembly in 2001 (effective 2003) and renamed the International Classification of Functioning, Disability and Health (ICF). This change reflected a more positive approach, minimizing marginalization and stigmatization by incorporating the concept of functioning (18, 19).

The ICF seeks to provide a standardized, reliable and cross-culturally applicable language to describe human functioning and disability as important elements of health, using positive language and a universal view of disability. This tool is invaluable because it provides the necessary building blocks for modeling and studying different aspects of functioning and disability. The ICF, being a classification of health, assumes the presence of a health condition of any kind, encompassing all aspects of health and some components of well-being relevant to health. This document offers a systematized coding scheme for application in various health information systems, a scientific basis for the study and understanding of health, levels of functioning and disability, as well as a common language with precise definitions that allow the comparison of information and facilitate communication between different professional disciplines and areas of knowledge (18, 19).

- Objectives of the ICF (20):
    - To provide a scientific basis for the study of health and related conditions, as well as for understanding their outcomes and determinants.
    - Establish a common language to describe health and related conditions, improving communication among health professionals, researchers, health policy makers, and the general population, including people with disabilities.
    - Allow comparison of data between countries, health disciplines, services and different points in time.
    - To provide a systematized coding system to be applied in health information systems.

The ICF has been accepted as one of the social classifications of the United Nations and incorporates the Standard Rules for the Equalization of Opportunities for Persons with Disabilities. It provides a conceptual framework applicable to personal health care, including prevention, health promotion and participation enhancement, removing social barriers and promoting the development of social supports and facilitators. The ICF classifies deficits resulting from a health condition, without regard to individual abilities. It includes health domains and categories that may not be relevant to the actual context of the individual or the needs of the assessor. It does not address essential personal factors in functional assessment, so it should be used globally and with clear objectives, not as a comprehensive instrument (20, 21).

- Personal factors: These factors include age, race, gender, physical fitness, personality, education, behavior and coping strategies. Although they may not be part of a health condition, they constitute the individual's life background. These factors are critical for physical therapists and rehabilitation teams to achieve their goals, but they can also present obstacles in the rehabilitation process.
- Organization of information: The ICF systematically groups a person's domains in relation to his or her health condition, describing what a person with a disorder or disease can do. Functioning is understood globally, encompassing bodily functions, activities and participation. Disability includes impairments, activity limitations and participation restrictions, with contextual factors interacting to particularize the disabling condition.
- ICF Structure: The ICF organizes the information into two parts: Functioning and Disability, and Contextual Factors. Each part has two components, and each component contains several domains and categories as classification units (20):
  - Functioning and Disability Components:
    - Body: Includes two classifications, one for body system functions (mental, sensory, pain, voice and speech, cardiovascular, hematological, immunological, digestive, metabolic, endocrine, respiratory, genitourinary, reproductive, neuromusculoskeletal and movement-related, skin functions and related structures) and one for body structures (anatomical parts such as organs, limbs and their components).
    - Activities and Participation: Covers the range of domains related to functioning from an individual (learning, knowledge application, communication, mobility, self-care) and social (participation in society, inclusion, etc.) perspective. Activity

limitations are difficulties in performing various activities, and participation restrictions are problems in engaging in life situations.

- Components of contextual factors:
    - Environmental factors: Affect all components of functioning and disability, organized from the immediate to the general environment. They include products and technology, natural environment and changes resulting from human activity, support and relationships, attitudes, services, systems and policies.
    - Personal factors: These constitute the particular background of an individual's life and lifestyle, including characteristics unrelated to a health condition (sex, race, other health status, physical fitness, lifestyles, habits, coping styles, social background, education, occupation, past and current experiences, behavioral patterns and personality). These factors, due to their great social and cultural variability, are not currently classified in the ICF.

The ICF systematically organizes and classifies the domains of health and disability, establishing relationships and interactions between the various components of health and functioning. Although it provides an important conceptual framework, it does not encompass all dimensions of human development or the broad spectrum of abilities that an individual may develop. Adaptation to disability depends on previous experiences and personal interpretation of life events, which determines the psychosocial impact and actual degree of disability.

7.3. Special considerations in the assessment of functional capacity.

Functional assessment is a process that involves the collection and analysis of information obtained through evaluation, the identification of problems and user needs, and the application of instruments to verify hypotheses and issue a functional diagnosis, prognosis and decision making. This process focuses on measuring the individual's abilities to perform functional activities, understood as tasks that make up normal and autonomous performance, taking into account the demands of the environment and society. It detects not only the individual's difficulties, but also his or her possibilities and potential to develop new skills, considering the interaction of personal and environmental factors. The functional prognosis depends on the clinical judgment obtained through the assessment, but also on contextual variables that affect the individual's daily life. Functional assessment should be comprehensive, continuous and dynamic, facilitating sound decisions. This assessment includes physical, mental, emotional and social aspects, and requires tools that cover multiple dimensions of functioning. Disability is manifested when the individual's performance does not meet social expectations, influenced by impairments in bodily functions or social barriers. The choice of assessment instruments depends on the clarity of the assessor about the information required, considering that functional activities are also a referential concept for the user, who identifies the activities essential to his or her well-being. Functional assessment should provide information for decision making, goal planning, interdisciplinary communication and optimization of the therapeutic intervention, ensuring the safety and effectiveness of the process. The competence of the assessor is crucial to organize, analyze and relate the information obtained, selecting the appropriate instruments according to the objectives and conditions of the individual (20, 21).

7.4. Functional capacity assessment scales.

The process of assessing functional capacity involves considering multiple aspects of the individual and his or her environment. Various methods are used to collect information, such as observation, interviews, self-assessment, surveys, and application of standard or non-standard instruments. The selection of instruments is based on the interpretation of the information obtained and should be consistent with the objectives of the assessment (22).

The objective of the application of these instruments is to measure the ability to perform activities independently, although they do not always accurately reflect all the capabilities and limitations of the individual. It is important to differentiate the factors that can cause impairments and disabilities, identify the main problems and establish the relationship between them. When choosing an instrument, the purpose of the assessment, the characteristics of the population or user, and the environment where the assessment is performed should be considered. It is also important to know the psychometric properties of the instruments, their sensitivity to detect significant changes and their specificity to be clinically or scientifically useful. There are several functional capacity assessment instruments, classified according to activities of daily living, instrumental activities of daily living and advanced activities for a satisfactory social life. Some of the most commonly used instruments include the Katz Index and the Barthel Scale for assessing basic activities of daily living, and the Lawton and Brody Scale for instrumental activities. Performance-based tests such as the Tinetti Scale are also used to assess balance and gait. These tests are not intended to rate limitations in prespecified activities, but to identify what the individual can perform in a specific situation (22).

The assessment of functional capacity is comprehensive and multidimensional, often requiring the application of several instruments depending on information needs. No single instrument addresses all aspects of human functioning or the individual's profile completely. The following are the functional capacity assessment scales.

For basic activities of daily living (BADL) we find:

- The Katz Index: This scale has been developed to evaluate stroke, elderly and multiple sclerosis patients. It is a tool used to assess a person's functional ability in six areas of basic activities of daily living. The score is assigned as follows (23, 24):
  - Independent: 1 point
  - Dependent: 0 point

	KATZ INDEX	Points
Bath	Independent: Bathes alone or requires assistance to wash an area, such as the back, or a disabled limb. Dependent: Requires assistance with washing more than one area, getting in or out of the bathtub, or is unable to bathe alone.	1 0
Dress	Independent: Takes clothes out of drawers and closets, puts them on, and buttons. The act of tying shoes is excluded. Dependent: Does not dress self, or remains partially undressed.	1 0

Use of WC	Independent: Goes to the toilet alone, fixes clothes and cleans himself.	1
	Dependent: Requires assistance to go to the toilet.	0
Transfers	Independent: Rises and lies in bed by self, and can get up from a chair by self.	1
	Dependent: Requires assistance to get up and lie down in bed or chair. Does not make one or more trips.	0
Continence	Independent: Complete control of urination and defecation.	1
	Dependent: Partial or total incontinence of urination or defecation.	0
Feeding	Independent: Brings food to the mouth from the plate or equivalent (cutting meat is excluded).	1
	Dependent: Requires assistance to eat, does not eat at all, or requires parenteral feeding.	0

Scoring:

A. Independent in feeding, continence, transfers, toilet use, dressing and bathing.
B. Independent in all but one (bathroom).
C. Independent in all but bathroom and one other function.
D. Independent in all but bathing, dressing and one other function.
E. Independent in all but bathing, dressing, toilet use and one other function.
F. Independent in all but bathing, dressing, toilet use, transfers and one other function.
G. Dependent in all functions
H. Dependent in at least two functions, but not classifiable as C, D, E or F.

Table 3. Evaluation of the Katz index (23,24).

- The Barthel Index: This is one of the most widely used scales today. It uses a scoring scale to assess functional ability in activities of daily living. Each activity is scored according to the degree of independence of the individual in that task, with a maximum score of 100. The allocation of points for each activity is shown below (23, 25):

BARTHEL'S INDEX		Points
Feeding	Totally independent	10
	Needs help to cut meat, bread, etc.	5
	Dependent	0
Bath	Independent. In and out of the bathroom alone	10

	Needs supervision or minimal assistance	5
	Dependent	0
Dress	Independent. Able to put on and take off clothes, button buttons, tie shoes, etc.	10
	Need help	5
	Dependent	0
Arrange	Independent to wash hands, comb hair, shave, apply make-up, etc.	10
	Supervision or assistance with shaving, make-up or hair styling, independent of others	5
	Dependent	0
Deposition	Continent	10
	Occasionally an episode of incontinence or need help in giving incontinent suppositories or enemas	5
	Incontinent	0
Urination	Continent or is able to care for the probe	10
	Occasionally, maximum of one episode of incontinence in 24 hours, need help to care for the catheter	5
	Incontinent	0
Use of restroom	Independent to go to the toilet, take off and put on clothes	10
	Needs help going to the bathroom, but cleans up after himself	5
	Dependent	0
Transfer armchair / bed	Independent for transfers	10
	Minimal physical assistance or supervision	5
	Dependent	0
Wandering	Independent. Walk only 50 meters.	10
	Needs physical assistance or supervision to walk 50 meters	5
	Dependent	0
Steps	Independent up and down stairs	10
	Needs physical assistance or supervision	5
	Dependent	0

Scoring:

- Total Dependent (less than 20 points)

- Severe Dependency (20 - 35 points)
- Moderate Dependency (40 - 55 points)
- Mild Dependency (greater than or equal to 60 points)
- Independence (100 points).

Table 4. Barthel index score (23, 25).

- Lawton and Brody: Another tool used to assess functional ability in activities of daily living. Unlike the Barthel Index, which focuses on basic activities such as personal grooming and feeding, the Lawton and Brody scale focuses on more complex instrumental activities that are necessary for independent living in the community (23,26).

LAWTON AND BRODY		Points
A. Ability to use the telephone	1. Uses the telephone on own initiative, looks up and dials numbers, etc.	1
	2. Dial a few well-known numbers	1
	3. Answers the phone, but does not dial	1
	4. Does not use the phone at all	0
B. Shopping	1.Make all necessary purchases independently.	1
	2. Buy small things independently	1
	3. You need company to make any purchase	0
	4. Completely unable to go shopping	0
C. Meal preparation	1. Plans, prepares and serves food properly and independently 2.	1
	2. Prepares appropriate meals if given the ingredients.	1
	3. Heats, serves, and prepares meals or prepares meals, but does not maintain an adequate diet.	0
	4. Needs to have food prepared and served.	0
D. Home Care	Takes care of the house alone or with occasional help (e.g., hard work) 2.	1
	2. Performs light housework such as washing dishes, making the bed, etc.	1
	3. Performs light housework, but is unable to maintain an acceptable level of cleanliness	0
	4. Needs help with all household chores	0
	5. Does not participate in any domestic chores	0
E. Laundry	1. Completely performs the personal laundry.	1
	2. Washes small clothes, socks, etc.	1

	3. You need someone else to do the washing.	0
F. Means of transportation	1. Travels independently in transport or drives own car	1
	2. Able to arrange your transportation by cabs, but not other transportation.	1
	3. Travels on public transport if accompanied by another person.	1
	4. Only travels by cab or car with the help of others.	0
	5. Does not travel at all	0
G. Responsibility for medication	1. Is responsible in the use of medication in the dosage and times indicated 2.	1
	2. Takes medication responsibly if it is prepared in separate doses.	0
	3. Is not able to take responsibility for his or her own medication.	0
H. Ability to use money	1. Handles financial matters independently (budgets, writes checks and invoices, goes to the bank) 1 collects and knows his income	1
	2. Manages day-to-day expenses, but needs help going to the bank and making large expenditures.	1
	3. Unable to handle money	0

Instrumental assessment of Lawton and Brody (23).

- Red Cross Physical Disability Scale: The Red Cross Physical Disability Scale, developed in this hospital in Madrid, was published a few years after the previous ones. It was initially designed for the assessment of chronic patients cared for at home and later its use was extended to the different hospital levels of geriatric services. It is the first Spanish scale and probably the most widely used in the country, mainly in geriatric units and nursing homes. It has abundant literature and is very easy to apply. It evaluates: activities of daily living, state assistance for ambulation, level of mobility restriction and sphincter continence. It quantifies the patient's disability in whole numbers, from 0 (independent) to 5 (maximum dependency). It has low interobserver reproducibility and presents good correlation with the Katz and Barthel indices. Its main limitations are the subjectivity in the interpretation of each grade, mainly in the intermediate ones (27).

In instrumental activities of daily living (IADL) scales are used to assess the patient's degree of adaptation to the environment and his or her ability to maintain independence not only at home but also in the community. IADLs depend on physical capacity and also, to a large extent, on the affective, cognitive and even social environment. Therefore, the items that assess them are not culturally neutral. An example of this is that in England "making a cup of tea" is included among them, which would make little sense in Spain for both women and men. For this reason, there are versions of scales that include adaptations.

- Modified Rapid Disability Rating Scale (RDRS-2): Used in the evaluation of patients with dementia. It evaluates functional and cognitive capacity in a fairly broad and rapid manner. It is a questionnaire with 18 questions divided into three sections. The first section evaluates eight activities of daily living such as eating, walking, dressing, transferring, ability to be in bed, and controlling incontinence. The second section measures aspects such as mobility and social interaction, while the third assesses neuropsychological behaviors such as cooperation and cognitive appraisal. The score ranges from 18 to 72 points; the higher the score, the greater the degree of disability (28).
- Pfeiffer's Functional Activities Questionnaire (FAQ): Created for dementia screening, it assesses eleven functional activities (IADLs) including money management, shopping, meal preparation, keeping up with community news, medication management or traveling alone. A score equal to or greater than 6 points alerts to a pathological deficit in IADLs due to dementia, physical disability, comorbidity or other cause. The assessment can be performed by the subject himself, but it is preferable that it is done by a close relative, because in normal subjects the reliability is high, but in people with cognitive impairment, this reliability is reduced (29).
- Lawton and Brody Instrumental Activities Scale: This scale assesses eight items: using the telephone, shopping, preparing meals, performing household chores, using public transportation, responsibility in taking medication and ability to handle money. It has good concurrent validity with other IADL scales and has served as a template for other scales. An unvalidated translation is available in Spanish (30).

By designing multidimensional tools, a more comprehensive and complex approach is pursued, integrating in capabilities such as gait, balance, community aspect and mental factors in addition to ABVD and AIBV.

- Tinetti Scale: The Tinetti Scale, also known as the Tinetti Performance Oriented Mobility Assessment (POMA), is a tool used to assess balance and gait in older adults. It consists of two main sections: one for balance and one for gait. The total score helps predict fall risk (31):

Tinetti Scale			
Part I: Equilibrium		**Points**	**Date**
Seated balance	Leans or slides in the chair	0	
	Firm and secure	1	
Get up	Incapable without assistance	0	
	Able to use arms as an aid	1	
	Able to stand up with an attempt	2	
Immediate equilibrium (5') when standing up	Unstable (wobbles, shifts feet, marked trunk swaying)	0	
	Stable, but uses walker, cane, crutches, or other supportive objects	1	
	Stable without the use of canes or other supports	2	
Standing balance	Unstable	0	
	Stable with increased bearing area (heels more than 10cm apart) or use a walker, gait trainer or other support.	1	
	Narrow support base without any support	2	
Push	Tends to fall off	0	
	Wobbles, holds on, but stands firm	1	
Eyes closed	Unstable	0	
	Stable	1	
360° rotation	Discontinuous steps	0	
	Continuous steps	1	
	Unstable (catches or wobbles)	0	
	Stable	1	
Sit	Insecure (miscalculates distance, falls into chair)	0	
	Uses arms or does not have a smooth movement	1	
	Safe, smooth movement	2	
Total balance: / 16			

Part II March		Points	Date
Start of the march	Hesitates, hesitates or makes multiple attempts to get started	0	
	Not hesitant	1	
Step length and height	Right foot does not overtake left foot with step in swing phase	0	
	The right foot is fully raised	1	
	Left foot does not overtake right foot with step in swing phase	0	
	The left foot overtakes the right foot with the right step.	1	
	The left foot does not lift completely off the ground with the step in the swing phase.	0	
	The left foot is fully raised	1	
Pitch symmetry	Step length with the right and left foot is different (estimated).	0	
	The steps are equal in length	1	
Continuity of steps	For or there is discontinuity between steps	0	
	The steps are continuous	1	
Trajectory	Accentuated deviation	0	
	Moderate or medium deviation or use of aids	1	
	Right without the use of aids	2	
Trunk	Marked swing or use aids	0	
	No rocking, but there is flexion of the knees, back or outward extension of the arms.	1	
	No rocking or bending, no use of aids	2	
Gait posture	Separated heels	0	
	Heels almost touching while walking	1	
Total gear: / 12			
Grand Total: / 28			

Table 6. Assessment of stability Tinetti Test (31).

- Functional independence measure (FIM): One of the most prominent in the field of recovery is the functional independence measure (FMI), designed to assess changes in the operative level over time and the achievements of the recovery process, using numerical indicators that reflect the degree of dependence or disability in relation to the amount and type of support needed by the individual. It is easy to use, accurate and reliable, and can be used by various specialists in the recovery team (32).

Since its creation, the FIM has been the most widely used and disseminated instrument in the scientific literature. It was created with the idea of creating a global disability measurement index similar to the Barthel index but with greater sensitivity and including the cognitive and psychosocial alterations that the Barthel index did not contemplate in patients with brain damage. It evaluates 18 items divided into six categories: personal care, sphincter control, mobility, locomotion, communication and social cognition, in relation to basic and instrumental activities of daily living. Each item can be evaluated at seven levels, from 1 (total assistance) to 7 (total independence), with a total score ranging from 18 (minimum) to 126 (maximum). For use in the Spanish population, there is a translated and adapted version (33, 34).

Functional Independence Measure (FMI)	**Level**
Self-care	
Feeding	
Personal grooming	
Bath	
Upper body dress	
Lower body dress	
Toilet	
Sphincter control	
Bladder control	
Bowel control	
Mobility, relocation	
Bed, chair, wheelchair	
Bathroom	
Bathtub, shower	
Ambulation	
Bed / wheelchair	
Stairs	
Communication	
Compression	
Expression	

Social knowledge	
Social interaction Troubleshooting Memory	
Total	
Functional Independence Measure (FMI) Levels	
7 complete independence 6 modified independence	**Without assistance**
Modified unit 5 monitoring 4 minimum attendance (subject to 75%) 3 moderate attendance (subject 50%) **Full dependency** 2 maximum attendance (subject 50%+) 1 total attendance	**With assistance**

Functional independence assessment (FMI) (32, 33).

- The SF-36 comprises 36 statements: It is made up of self-assessed performance-based statements that constitute eight distinct scales: physical ability, social integration, task performance, psychological well-being, vitality/fatigue, discomfort, and general health perceptions. The questions can have nominal or ordinal responses, with each response being assigned a score on each scale. These scores are summed and transformed to obtain a percentage; 100% represents optimal health status. This resource has been used in numerous studies describing health status and physical fitness in users with various limitations. High reliability and validity have been evidenced (35).
- Outcomes and Assessment Information Set (OASIS): Designed to collect data in adult home care services to determine the quality of care and establish outcomes. The current version of the OASIS (OASIS-B) includes 79 statements that address social, environmental, social support, health status, and functioning. It does not constitute a functional assessment in itself; it should be integrated into the clinical record to highlight various aspects of a user's condition with specific

needs. The OASIS was developed as part of a research program, over more than 10 years. It has been field-tested through projects and demonstrations since 1999, and it is a requirement for home care entities to participate in the Health Care Financing Administration program (36, 37).

- Pediatric Evaluation of Disability Inventory (PEDI): It was developed to assess the functional ability of children between 6 months and 7.5 years, including those with physical disabilities. Originally created for the functional evaluation of young children, it can also be used to evaluate older children whose functional abilities are below what is expected for a 7.5 year old child without disability. It measures both ability and performance of functional activities in three areas: self-care, mobility, and social function, through three scales: functional abilities (197 items), caregiver assistance (20 items), and need for modifications (20 items) (38).
- Rosow-Breslau Scale: Widely used in the field of geriatrics, it seeks to detect limitations in performing a series of daily activities that can be associated with functional dependence. The activities assessed are the ability to walk 800 meters without assistance and without stopping; the ability to walk up and down stairs without assistance; and the ability to perform work at home, such as cleaning walls or gardening activities (39).
- Nagi scale: The items of this scale are more heterogeneous (raising the arms above the head, handling small objects, lifting weights of about 5 kg or large, bending, squatting, kneeling and standing). Some studies have specifically assessed advanced functional activities of daily living including recreational, sporting or cultural activities such as running, swimming, sport walking or hunting and fishing (40).

Other specific scales that we can use according to different pathologies are:

For stroke evaluation we found:

- Modified Rankin Scale: It is used for clinical practice and evaluates physical disability after stroke. It is divided into 7 levels, from 0 (no symptoms) to 6 (death). It is one of the most widely used scales, but it is not free of discrepancies among professionals when evaluating the same patient. To avoid this variability, a structured interview is recommended (41,42).

- Frenchay Activities Index: Created for use in stroke patients to analyze their social and instrumental functions of daily living. It assesses patients' ability to perform complex activities related to home maintenance, leisure, hobbies and social interaction. It consists of 15 items with a score from 1 to 4 for each item. Its overall value ranges from a minimum of 15 (inactive subject) to a maximum of 60 points (very active person). The frequency of each activity or task during the last three to six months is also considered. It can be administered by a therapist or by the patient himself in an estimated time of 5 minutes (43).

For multiple sclerosis:

- Multiple Sclerosis Impact Scale: It is a self-report measure consisting of 29 items grouped into two subscales: 20 items associated with a physical scale and 9 items associated with a psychological scale. The items have five response options, from 1 (not at all) to 5 (extremely). The scoring range is from 0 to 100, where 100 indicates a greater impact of the disease on daily function (worse health status). Its use is increasingly widespread and it has been translated into more than 20 languages, including Spanish (44).
- Expanded Disability Status Scale: This is a widely used procedure, despite its insufficient validity and reliability, in the functional assessment of multiple sclerosis. It provides a total score on a scale ranging from 0 to 10. The first levels, from 1.0 to 4.5, refer to people with a high degree of ambulatory ability, while levels 5.0 to 9.5 refer to loss of ambulatory ability. Level 10 refers to death caused by the disease (45).

In Amyotrophic Lateral Sclerosis (ALS)

- Revised Amyotrophic Lateral Sclerosis Functional Rating Scale: This is one of the most clinically used instruments to assess disease progression. It consists of 12 items grouped into 4 dimensions (fine mobility, broad mobility, bulbar function and respiratory function) that grade disabilities in activities of daily living. It is a validated scale widely used in clinical trials, but due to cultural differences it has been necessary to adapt it for the Spanish population. This Spanish version is a highly reliable and valid tool for the functional assessment of Spanish patients affected by ALS (46).

For Parkinson's evaluation, we found:

- Schwab and England Activities of Daily Living: By means of an interview, it evaluates the patient's global functional capacity and degree of dependence in relation to motor aspects of Parkinson's disease. The score is expressed as a percentage, from 0 (normal state) to 100 (bedridden and vegetative impairment). It is a scale widely used in clinical practice and research, but may present some problems in its application due to the lack of standardization and the fact that it does not take into account certain characteristic aspects of this disease, such as dyskinesias and non-motor symptoms (47).

To go beyond the purpose of functional capacity assessment, health professionals should not lose sight of the fact that this process should always be framed in the daily reality of the individual. It is crucial that the user understands why he/she faces difficulties in performing a functional task or activity, what are the possibilities of overcoming these difficulties, how this affects his/her lifestyle, role performance and relationships with his/her environment. Decision-making should arise from a dynamic and positive interaction between the evaluator and the user, and from an understandable communication through an accessible and everyday language, to establish an authentic therapeutic relationship, in which the physiotherapist and the user interact, each one from his knowledge, experience and capabilities, to achieve goals set together. In this way, the best path to functional recovery or the reconstruction of a satisfactory lifestyle is found (37).

8. Analytical evaluation methods in physical therapy.

8.1. Concept and classification.

Analytical assessment is a process that studies the different structures of the organism in isolation, without establishing relationships between them, and constantly refers to their behavior in a normal state. This process looks for signs that indicate alterations in the normal structure and function (7).

In physiotherapy, the analytical assessment includes at least the examination of the integumentary system, joints, muscles and nervous system. Depending on the pathology, more specific assessments can be added, such as respiratory assessment. The methods used in the analytical assessment are (7):

- Visual: Observation.
- Manual: Palpation and mobilization of different tissues.
- Instrumental: Measurement of physical magnitudes, recording of their variations and comparison with normality standards.

8.2. Examination of the integumentary system.

The integumentary system, consisting of the skin and its appendages, covers the entire surface of the human body. Its importance lies in its multiple vital functions and its influence on the ability to move. In addition to its structural relevance, the skin plays a crucial social role by facilitating interaction with the environment, the perception of sensations and the expression of emotions. Understanding the structure and function of the integumentary system is essential for health care professionals in the assessment of human body function and movement. Impairments in this system may be due to direct alterations or to various health conditions. Peripheral vascular diseases, sensory impairments, alterations in consciousness and long periods in bed without postural changes can affect the skin. Therefore, physical therapists should perform a thorough examination of the integumentary system to determine its current condition and its impact on other body structures, motor skills, and the patient's social participation (48).

8.2.1. Anatomophysiological and biomechanical considerations of the integumentary system.

The skin, the most extensive and superficial organ of the human body, plays a crucial role in medical evaluation by reflecting a person's overall health.

- Main functions of the skin (48):
  - Protection: Acts as a barrier against physical, chemical and biological agents.
  - Thermal Regulation: Controls temperature through sweating and blood circulation in the dermis.
  - Sensory Communication: Allows the perception of sensations such as touch, pressure, temperature and pain.
  - Elimination and absorption: Excretes salts, ammonia, urea and other substances through sweat, in addition to absorbing chemicals and gases.
  - Vitamin D synthesis: Generated by exposure to the sun's UV rays.
  - Self-repair: Facilitates wound healing through cell division.
  - Cosmetic Appearance: Defines personal identity.

- Skin structure (48):
  - Epidermis: The most superficial layer, composed of keratinocytes that provide thermal, biological and chemical protection. Also includes melanocytes and immune cells.
  - Dermis: The deepest and most vascularized layer, it contains collagen, elastic and reticular fibers that give it strength and elasticity. It houses hair follicles, sweat and sebaceous glands, and numerous nerve endings.
  - Hypodermis (Subcutaneous Tissue): Stores adipose tissue, anchors the dermis and connects to deeper structures, aiding in heat conservation and as an energy reserve.

- Skin adnexa (48):
  - Hair: Provides protection and participates in thermal and sensory regulation. Its characteristics vary according to breed, sex and genetics.
  - Nails: Formed by keratin, they help in gripping and provide protection to the fingertips.

- Sweat glands: They regulate body temperature through the excretion of sweat. There are two types: eccrine (present in almost all skin) and apocrine (in armpits and genital areas).
- Sebaceous glands: Produce sebum to keep skin and hair supple and conserve body heat.

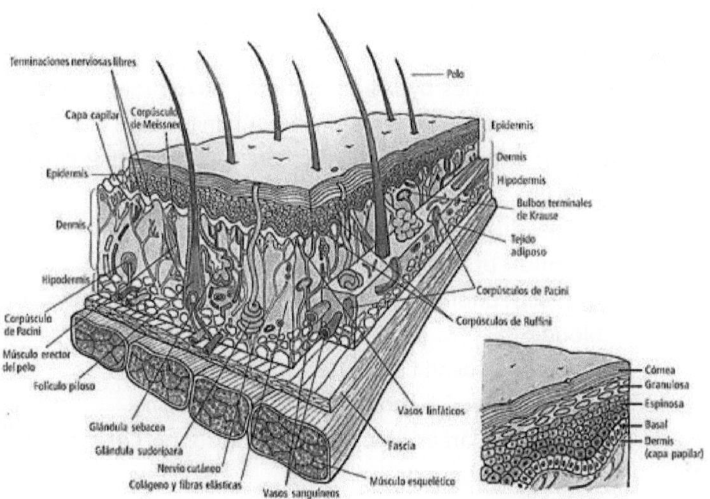

Figure 8. Anatomical structure of the skin (8).

- Clinical Significance (48): The skin is crucial in the functional assessment of human body movement. Deficiencies in the skin may indicate underlying health problems, such as peripheral vascular disease or sensory problems. Therefore, it is essential for physical therapists to perform a thorough examination of the integumentary system to assess its condition and its impact on other structures and functions of the body.

8.2.2. Interview and review of the integumentary system.

The evaluation of the integumentary system includes the interview and health history of the user, together with a thorough review of the system and the application of specific tests. The recording of information should be detailed, both qualitatively and quantitatively. If deficiencies of the skin and its attachments are identified that affect the user's activity and participation, it is essential to document the causes in order to design an appropriate therapeutic program. During the interview, possible structural skin deficiencies (bedsores, ulcers, rashes, etc.) should be investigated and, if present, asked about their size and location. It is also relevant to inquire about sensory deficits, activity limitations, use of orthopedic aids, medications and physical aids administered (49).

- Valuation Phases (49):
  - Inspection:
    - Skin color: Varies by breed and may have areas of increased pigmentation due to sun exposure. Changes such as:
      - Pallor: whitish or marbled coloration, indicating circulatory deficit.
      - Redness: May indicate hypervascularization, inflammation or the onset of eschar in supportive areas.
      - Cyanosis: poor venous return, insufficient oxygenation of the blood.
      - Blackening: dead tissue, necrotized areas.
      - Blue or yellowish spots: Ecchymosis, bruising.
      - Dark brown areas: Hyperkeratosis in support areas.
    - Skin appearance:
      - Peeling: Frequent after prolonged immobilization with plaster or skin diseases such as psoriasis.
      - Cracks or stretch marks: In areas of tension or after sudden changes in weight.
      - Orange peel: Indicates alteration of the connective tissue, cellulite.
    - Examination of the scalp: Alterations in hairiness or dry, brittle nails may indicate a vascular disorder.
    - Thickness: Thin, hairy skin covers most of the body, while thick, non-hairy skin is found on palms and soles. Variations may indicate vascular or systemic deficiencies.
    - Skin tissue volume: Differences in volume may be related to edema, affecting the biomechanical properties of the skin. We can find:
      - Edema: Infiltration and stagnation of liquids in the subcutaneous tissues, predominantly distal.
      - Inflammation: Local disposition, circumscribed to the lesion area.

    - Trophic condition of hair and nails: Dry and brittle hair and nails with deformities provide information on nutritional deficiencies and systemic diseases.
    - Presence of wounds and scars: Especially in areas close to a joint, where they can limit joint mobility.

- Palpation and Tissue Mobilization:
    - Temperature, humidity and texture: Palpate the skin with the dorsal surface of the hand to assess temperature; changes indicate vascular deficiencies, infection or inflammation.
    - Consistency and elasticity: Normal skin is smooth, soft and uniform. Changes may indicate cysts, scars or thickening.
    - Mobility and flexibility: Move the skin to identify adhesions to deep tissues. Evaluate consistency, extensibility, elasticity, flexibility, viscoelasticity and rigidity.
    - Identification of pain and edema: Palpate painful areas to determine the cause. Assess the origin of edema (venous or lymphatic) and its relation to the mechanical properties of the skin.
    - Turgor: Assess turgor through the formation of folds; delay in the return to the initial position indicates aging, dehydration or edema.

8.3. Manual valuation

- Assessment of the mechanical properties of the skin (10):
    - Skin fold: A pinch of skin is taken between the fingers. Ease of detachment indicates extensibility, and rapid return to its position indicates elasticity. Alterations such as dehydration or edema may leave a residual fold.

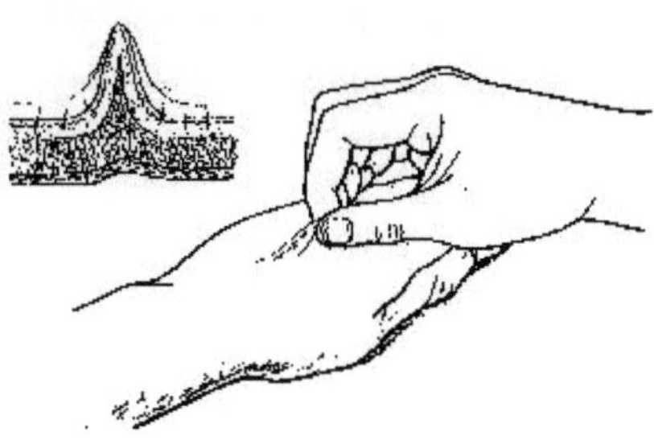

Figure 9. Assessment by skinfold (8).

- Rolled pinch: Assesses the mobility of the skin with respect to the underlying tissues and may reveal painful cellulagic areas.
- Transverse friction: Detects hypomobile areas or adhesions to deep planes.
- Wounds and scars: Assess mobility and elasticity to identify pathological scars (adherent, retractile, hypertrophic, keloid).
- Skin temperature: Assessed with the back of the hand. A localized increase may indicate inflammation, while a cooler area may suggest a circulatory deficit or trophic disorder.
- Sign of the fovea: Differentiates the origin of the edema: venous (retains the imprint after pressing with the finger) or lymphatic (does not retain the imprint).
- Peripheral pulses: Evaluation of the presence, absence and frequency of pulses.

8.4. Instrumental evaluation

Instrumentation is a crucial phase in the evaluation of the integumentary system, allowing the physical therapist to obtain accurate data on various qualities of the skin and underlying tissues. The main devices and methods used are described below:

- Tape measurement of limb circumference: Tape measure measurement is used to determine the perimeter of different body segments. This technique is especially useful for quantifying atrophies, edema and swelling that may be present in the extremities. To ensure accuracy and comparability of measurements over time it is essential to use constant reference points on the body such as bony reliefs. For example, when measuring arm circumference, a point 10 centimeters below the acromion can be used as a reference, while a point 15 centimeters above the upper edge of the patella can be used to measure thigh circumference. These references allow measurements to be consistent and comparable in future evaluations (50).

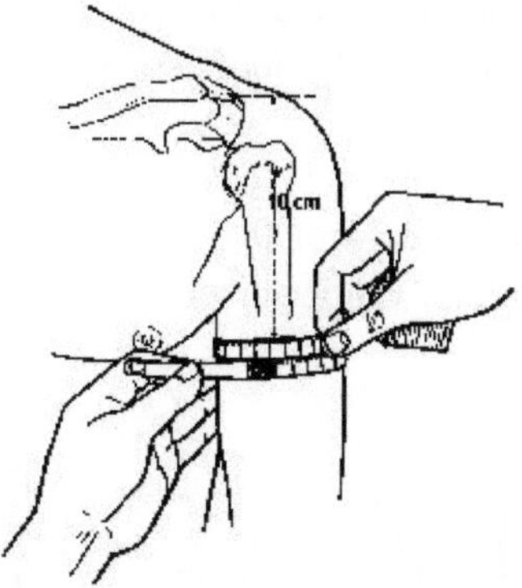

Figure 10. Measurement with tape measure of the arm perimeter (8).

- Volumetric measurement of a limb by Archimedes principle: The volumetric measurement is used to accurately quantify the magnitude of atrophies, edema and swelling in body segments where perimeter measurements are complex due to anatomical characteristics. A water tank equipped with a drainage tube is used for this measurement. When the affected limb is immersed in the tank, the displaced water is collected in a collection container and the volume in milliliters is recorded. To ensure the accuracy of the data it is crucial that the limb is always immersed to the same height for each test. In addition, the temperature of the water must be kept constant at each measurement since temperature variations can affect the volume of water displaced. These procedures ensure that the data obtained are accurate and comparable over time (51).

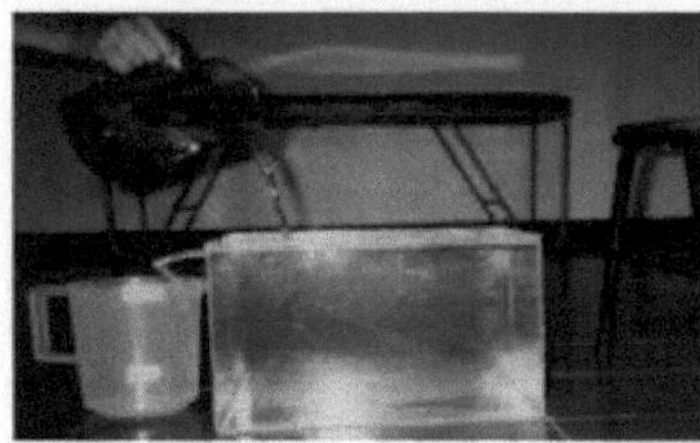
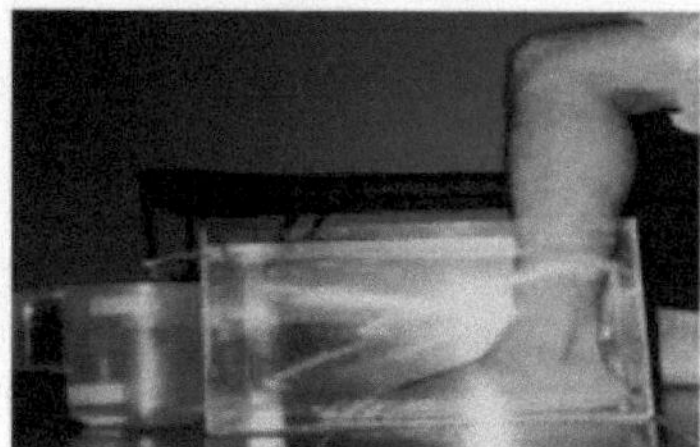

Figure 11. Volumetric measurement of the ankle and foot (51).

- Plicometer: The plicometer is used to measure the thickness of skin folds, making it possible to quantify the amount of adipose tissue and evaluate the trophic quality of the skin. This instrument consists of two articulated arms with blunt or flat ends to avoid unpleasant sensations during the measurement. It is preferable to use plicometers that maintain a constant pressure to guarantee the accuracy of the data, avoiding variations. In the absence of a plicometer, a Vernier caliper or vernier vernier can be used as an alternative (52).

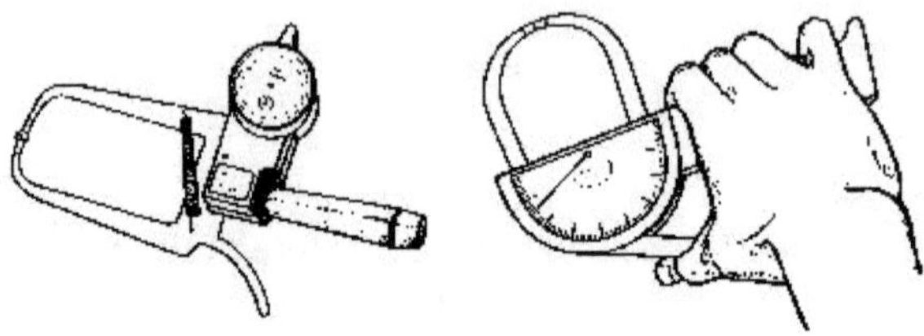

Figure 12. Measurement with plicometer (8).

- Footprint scanning by podoscope: The podoscope is used to detect abnormal footpad points on the sole of the foot and to differentiate the areas that bear more or less pressure. This method is crucial for identifying load distribution problems in the feet, providing valuable information for posture correction and injury prevention (53).

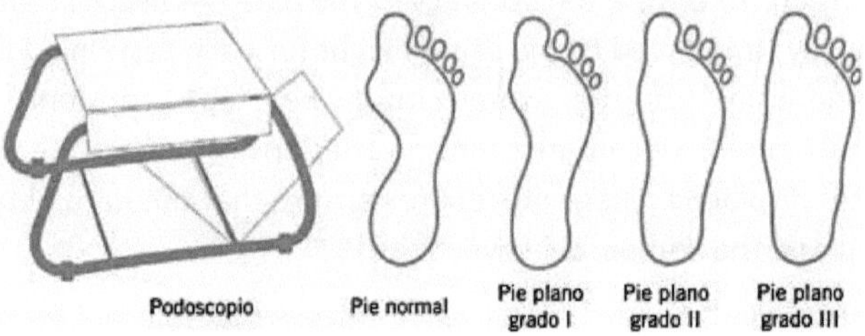

Figure 13. Podoscope and podogram with the degrees of flatfoot (53).

- The Möberg test: Involves staining with ninhydrin of the skin print collected on paper to evaluate the secretion of the sweat glands. This test provides information on the trophism of the area studied, helping to identify possible dysfunctions in sweating and the general state of the skin (54).
- Digital camera: The digital camera is an essential tool for documenting the evolution of cutaneous structural deficiencies. The photographs

are recorded in the user's health history, making it possible to objectively assess the effectiveness of the therapeutic plan or the natural evolution of the deficiencies. This visual documentation is crucial for detailed and accurate follow-up (55).

- Support Zone Glass: Support Zone Glass is used to identify areas of increased skin contact in a specific body region. A polished glass is placed over the area of interest, allowing the areas that bear the most pressure to be observed and located. This method is inexpensive and useful for identifying pressure areas, although more accurate technological devices are available (50).
- Sensitivity testing materials: Sensitivity testing requires a variety of materials, including a pin or paper clip, capped test tubes, a camel hair brush, a piece of cardboard or disposable facial tissue, common items such as keys, coins and pencils, small weights of equal size to gradually increase the weight, and samples of materials of different textures such as cotton, wool and silk. Additionally, a tuning fork and headphones are used to reduce ambient noise and focus the evaluation. The purpose and procedure of the sensitivity assessment is to identify the integrity of the nervous system, the type and degree of sensory impairment, and to delineate the body surface area involved. Superficial, deep or proprioceptive, and mixed or cortical sensibility are explored. For this purpose, dermatome maps are used to identify deficiencies in segmental cutaneous innervation. These maps serve as a guide to accurately locate and record the affected areas, facilitating diagnosis and planning of appropriate treatment (56).

9. Analytical joint assessment

A joint is the union of two bony ends. As mentioned in the previous section, joints are the axis of rotation about which angular movement is generated, i.e. the displacement of the bony lever thanks to muscular action. Joint levers allow a certain degree of freedom of movement in a plane and around an axis, depending on the joint morphology, the fulcrum and the existence of muscles that produce the movement. In addition to facilitating movement, joints transform shear forces (which can be damaging) into tensile forces (absorbed by periarticular soft tissues) and compressive forces (absorbed by bone and cartilage tissue) (57, 58).

9.1. Analytical evaluation of joints

The evaluation will be based on observation and palpation of the joint, as well as manual and instrumental assessment of its mobility. Before the assessment, it is essential to take into account the different types of joints. The following is a description of the different types of joints according to their capacity for movement and the presence or absence of synovium (57, 58):

9.1.1. Non-synovial or solid joints:

Non-synovial, or solid, joints are those in which the bony surfaces are joined by fibrous connective tissue or cartilage (usually fibrocartilage). These joints allow minimal movement (57, 58).

- Synarthrosis: Joints with a high degree of firmness and minimal range of motion. The bones are held together by irregular and dense connective tissue. These joints transmit and dissipate forces between the bones, reducing the possibility of injury. They are divided into:
  - Gonphosis: Union between the teeth and the adjacent bone, with the periodontal ligament interposed between them.
  - Sutures: Also known as sinfibrosis, they are the union between the bones of the skull, connected by a thin layer of connective tissue called sutural ligament. They are classified as:
    - Serrata or serrated suture: Serrated or toothed edges.
    - Squamous suture: Beveled edges.
    - Flat or harmonic suture: Flattened or rounded edges.
    - Schindelesis; A ridge-like surface that fits into a groove.

- Syndesmosis: Joints with a large amount of fibrous connective tissue that does not allow movement. Example: lower tibio-peroneal syndesmosis.
- Epiphyseal laminae of the growth plates: junction between the growth plate between the epiphysis and the metaphysis of long bones.
- Schindylesis: The surface of one bone fits into the groove of the other bone forming the joint. Example: the vomer bone fits into the groove of the sphenoid.

- Amphiarthrosis: Semi-mobile joints, with a significant level of firmness and some degree of mobility. The articular surfaces are flat or slightly concave and are covered with hyaline cartilage. They always have a fibrocartilage interosseous ligament that joins both articular surfaces and peripheral ligaments that reinforce the union between the bones. Example: joints between vertebral bodies (57, 58).
  - Symphysis: union of two bones by cartilage, usually located in the midline. Example: the symphysis pubis.
  - Synchondrosis: Joints that allow very little movement and may disappear with aging. Examples: the junction between the vertebral disc and adjacent vertebrae, the sphenobasilar joint and the xipho-sternal joints.

9.1.2. Synovial joints or diarthrosis.

Synovial joints are separated by a joint cavity filled with synovial fluid. The articular surfaces are covered by cartilage, usually of hyaline type, which prevents the bony ends from being in contact. This cartilage is aneural and avascular, so its nutrition is produced by imbibition, and in case of immobilization, it can lose mass, volume and resistance. These joints are covered by a joint capsule, composed of the synovial membrane on the inner side and the fibrous membrane (dense irregular connective tissue composed mainly of type I collagen fibers) on the outer side. Joint stability is reinforced by ligaments, which can be (57, 58):

- Intracapsular: Inside the capsule, but outside the synovial cavity, such as the anterior cruciate ligament of the knee.
- Extraarticular: Outside the joint capsule.

All synovial joints have proprioceptors, blood vessels and sensory nerves. In some cases, they may contain articular discs or menisci (usually fibrocartilaginous), peripheral impingements, fat pads and synovial folds. These elements increase joint congruence, improve the arc of motion and optimize load distribution. These joints can be classified according to their degrees of motion and the shape of the articular surfaces (57, 58):

- One degree of freedom:
    - Trochlear joint: One articular facet is shaped like a pulley, while the other is divided by a ridge that fits into the throat of the pulley. It only allows movement in the sagittal plane. Examples include the elbow, ankle and interphalangeal joints.
    - Trochoid joint: The articular surfaces are cylindrical, allowing only rotational movements in the horizontal plane. Examples are the proximal and distal radioulnar, costotransverse and atlantoaxial joints.
- Two degrees of freedom:
    - Condylar joint: Composed of two ellipsoids, spheres or ovoids, one surface is convex and the other concave. They can develop movement in the sagittal and frontal planes. Examples are the wrist, metacarpophalangeal and metatarsophalangeal joints, and the occipitoatloid joint.
    - Reciprocal socket: The articular surfaces are concave in one direction and convex in the other, allowing movements in the sagittal and frontal planes. Articular laxity may allow a third movement. Examples include the trapezometacarpal, sternocostoclavicular and calcaneocuboid joints.
- Three degrees of freedom:
    - Enarthrosis: Solid convex sphere that fits inside a concave surface, surrounded by powerful ligaments and muscles. They may experience a phenomenon called Codman's paradox. Examples are the glenohumeral, coxofemoral and astragaloescaphoid joints.
    - Arthrodias: The articular surfaces are flat and allow sliding movements of small amplitude. Some examples are the acromioclavicular, subtalar, tibioperoneal, costovertebral, and carpal and tarsal bone joints.

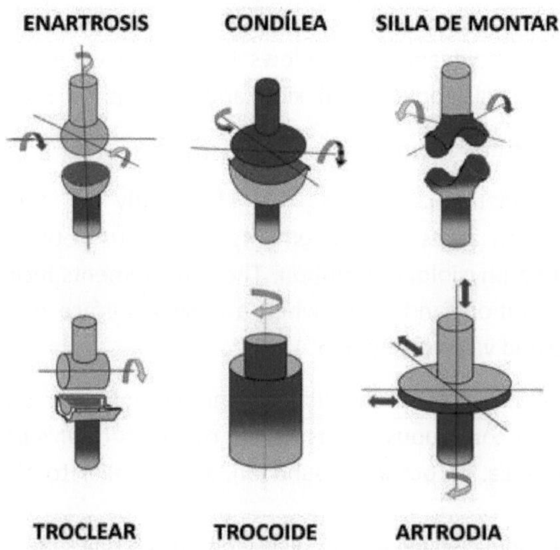

Figure 14. Types of diarthrosis joints (58).

9.1.3. Sinsarcosis

Sinsarcosis, often referred to as a "false joint," is a special type of joint between musculoskeletal structures that lacks articular cartilage. Rather than relying on cartilaginous articular surfaces, sinsarcosis relies on the interaction between muscles and the skeleton to allow for movement and stability. Although sinsarcosis lacks the typical structure of a joint, it is still crucial to the function and mobility of the human body. These musculoskeletal joints provide stability and control during movement, thus contributing to the health and functionality of the musculoskeletal system (57, 58).

A prominent example of sinsarcosis is the scapulothoracic joint. In this joint, the scapula (shoulder blade) is attached to the thorax by a series of muscles that insert into the scapula and originate from the ribs and spine. These muscles, such as the serratus anterior and the trapezius and rhomboid muscles, work together to allow a wide range of movement of the scapula, such as elevation, retraction and rotation, thus contributing to the mobility of the shoulder. Another example is the subdeltoid joint, where the deltoid muscle inserts on the top of the humerus and is attached to the underside of the acromion of the scapula. Although technically there is no true joint at this point, the interaction between the deltoid and bone allows for a wide variety of shoulder movements, such as abduction, flexion, and rotation (57, 58).

9.2. Arthrokinematics

Arthrokinematics focuses on the study of the intimate, fundamental and accessory movements that occur between articular surfaces during physiological motion. These movements include rolling, sliding and rotation, and occur when a convex surface moves over a concave one and vice versa (59, 60):

- Bearing: A movement in which contiguous points of one articular surface face contiguous points of the other articular surface at the same distance. It occurs around an axis parallel to the articular surface.
- Axis-free gliding: Involves the displacement of one articular surface over another, so that each point of one surface touches successive points of the other without repeating any of them. The axis of motion is parallel to the articular surface.
- Rotation or sliding with axis: It is the primary articular rotation when the longitudinal axis of the bone is perpendicular to the articular surface of the other articular segment.

These movements are often combined in joints where one surface is concave and the other convex, which changes the axis of rotation throughout the movement. Katelborn's concave-convex rule dictates that the direction of movements is defined by the shape of the articular surfaces (59, 60).

9.2.1. Functional Coefficient of Joint Mobility

The arc of motion represents the range of joint movement in degrees in the different planes of space. It is classified as active, active-assisted or passive. Often, joints allow a greater range of motion than is necessary for daily activities, so Rocher introduced the concept of "useful sector" of joint mobility or useful angle. According to this principle, a restriction of motion beyond the useful sector does not affect function, but a limitation within this sector, even a small one, can be very disabling (59).

The functional mobility coefficient is calculated by evaluating each movement in daily life and determining which arcs or angles are most useful or frequently used in normal activity. A higher coefficient is assigned to the angles of the useful sector that are more favorable for function. Rocher developed a table with these coefficients, where the mobility angle is multiplied by its corresponding coefficient to obtain the functional joint mobility coefficient. The maximum score is 100, corresponding to the ideal coefficient. In general, the first 15° of flexion from neutral position have a higher functional value than the next 15°, which translates into a higher mobility coefficient (59).

FUNCTIONAL JOINT MOBILITY COEFFICIENT		
FLEXION	0-30°	0,6
	30-75°	0,3
	75-180°	0,2
EXTENSION	0-30°	0,9
	30-80°	0,3
	>80°	0,1
ABD / ADD	0-180°	0,2

Table 8. Table of functional coefficient of joint mobility according to Rocher (59).

9.3. Joint observation

The articular examination should precede the examination of the corresponding cutaneous and subcutaneous tissue, as detailed in the previous point. Aspects to evaluate during the articular observation (61):

- Spontaneous Attitude of the Articulation:
    - Malformations or Pathological Sequelae: For example, flexum or recurvatum of the elbow, genu valgum or varus.
    - Antalgic Attitudes: Positions adopted to avoid pain.
    - Abnormal Postural Habits: For example, asthenic habitus with dorsal kyphosis, shoulder rolls and anterior cephalic projection.

- Volume increases: Indicators of pathologies such as synovial effusion, hemarthrosis, periarticular edema or joint inflammation are sought.
- Abnormal Bony Eminences: A comparison is made with the opposite side of the joint to detect osteophytes, fracture sequelae (such as misaligned fragments or hypertrophic fracture calluses) or amyotrophy highlighting bony eminences.

9.4. Joint palpation

Joint palpation is an essential part of the clinical examination, although it is considered a subjective procedure. Its purpose is to identify and evaluate various structures around the joints, detecting possible abnormalities or points of pain that may indicate pathology. The key aspects to consider during joint palpation are described below (61):

- Joint interlining: The joint interlining is the area of juxtaposition of the two bony epiphyses of a joint. It can be palpated through the joint capsule in most superficial joints. Its location usually coincides with the flexion skin folds, which facilitates its identification. However, in very deeply located joints, such as the coxofemoral joint, direct palpation of the interlining is not possible due to the depth of the structure.
- Periarticular bony prominences: The periarticular bony prominences are key areas for palpation as they coincide with muscle and ligament insertion zones. Palpation of these prominences allows assessment of the integrity of the muscle and ligament insertions. Any irregularities, such as the growth of osteophytes or changes due to misaligned fractures, may indicate pathological alterations.
- Ligaments: Ligament palpation is performed by a frictional motion perpendicular to the direction of the ligament fibers, which are previously placed in tension to facilitate localization. This method makes it possible to evaluate the integrity of the ligament and to detect any thickening, area of pain or abnormality that may be present.
- Tendons: It is essential to distinguish between tendons and ligaments during palpation. Unlike ligaments, tendons can be mobilized transversely between two fingers and are affected by the state of muscle contraction. Palpation of tendons allows identification of sore

spots, nodules, thickening or adhesions, providing crucial information about possible tendon pathologies.

It is convenient to perform palpation at the end of the clinical examination. The main reason is that a pain provoked by palpation could modify the patient's response and affect the results of other tests in the study. By evaluating the joint for the last time, it is ensured that any induced pain does not influence the accuracy of the previous observations.

9.5. Manual assessment of joint mobility

The joint mobility test aims to assess both qualitatively and quantitatively the different movements of the joint under examination, and to determine the articular causes that may be the origin of a limitation or increase of these movements. In order to focus exclusively on the articular factors involved in movement, it is crucial to perform the examination passively, since active movement simultaneously evaluates neurological and muscular factors:

- Joint limitations and hypermobility: Joint movement limitations, or hypomobilities, may be due to mechanical pathology, myofascial dysfunction and pericapsular alterations, among others. On the other hand, hypermobility is usually caused by alterations of the muscular or capsuloligamentous system, which generates joint instability and may hinder the maintenance of joint congruency. In general terms, the active assessment focuses on exploring the contractile (muscular) structures, while the passive assessment, in a state of muscular relaxation, preferentially studies the non-contractile structures (ligaments, tendons, capsules). Comparing the results of both assessments allows a differential diagnosis to be established (61, 62).
- Comparison and assessment conditions: The data obtained in the assessment should be compared with those of the contralateral limb or, if this is not possible, with the usual values observed in healthy subjects. It is essential to always perform the assessment under reproducible conditions. First, the passive degrees of freedom of the joint are evaluated by means of non-physiological movements: sliding, rolling, axial rotations, joint compression and decoaptation. This is done starting from positions where the muscular and

capsuloligamentous structures are distended, so as not to interfere with these movements (61, 62).

- Pain and functional deficiencies: If pain appears during compression, the cause is found in an intra-articular element (synovial fluid, cartilage, meniscus); if pain occurs during decoaptation, it is produced by periarticular soft tissues (ligaments, capsule). During passive assessment, it is important to avoid the Charcot reflex, where a violent or painful movement provokes an automatic protective contraction of the joint (61, 62).
- Objectives of the passive joint mobility test: Determine the characteristics and quality of movement: continuity, resistance, freedom, restrictions, hypomobility, hypermobility, etc. Relate pain or other impairments to the degrees of movement at which they appear and disappear. Recognize the causes of functional impairment by exploring the final sensation.
- Assessment of the active degrees of freedom: Next, the active degrees of freedom, those subject to voluntary control, are assessed. It is important to pay attention to the position of the supra and underlying joints so that the polyarticular muscles crossing the joint under study are in a shortened position and do not limit mobility. Several situations can be found (61, 62)
  - Temporary joint block: as in the case of meniscal lesions in the knee.
  - Joint stiffness or ankylosis: a total absence of mobility of a permanent nature.
  - Synostosis: limitation of mobility caused by the fusion of two bones by ossification of the connective tissue that joins them.
  - Partial limitation of symmetrical mobility: free mobility in the middle sector, but limited at both ends of the arc of motion.
  - Partial asymmetric mobility limitation: loss of amplitude affects only one end of the arc of motion, with physiological amplitude in the other direction.
- Terminal sensation of the movement: The terminal sensation of the movement or stop may be (62):
  - Dura or bony stop: contact between bony parts (e.g. in elbow extension). If it appears abnormally, it may indicate osteophytes, paraosteoarthropathies, hypertrophic fracture calluses, etc.

- Elastic: tensioning of the capsuloligamentary structures (e.g. in knee extension). May indicate retractile capsulitis or muscle retractions.
- Soft: contact of muscle masses (e.g., in elbow flexion). It also appears in acute hydrarthrosis or bursitis.
- "Razor-sharp": resistance that increases to a maximum and then suddenly gives way, typical in spasticity.
- Vacuum: stop before reaching resistance, due to intense pain.

- Articular Movement Barriers: In osteopathy, motor barriers are identified (62):
  - Physiological motor barrier (BMF): normal limitation during active movement due to soft tissue tension.
  - Elastic motor barrier (EMB): additional amplitude achieved passively after BMF, limited by the extensibility of ligaments and joint capsule.
  - Anatomical motor barrier (AMB): contact of bony surfaces, overcoming it causes injury.
  - Pathological barrier or restriction (BMP): abnormal limitation of movement due to various causes such as a muscular obstacle due to decreased muscle elasticity, which generates elastic resistance. A restriction by an articular surface, which is abrupt and hard, similar to the sensation of BPM, but which occurs earlier than expected. If the cause is a ligament or capsule, the sensation will be of a physiological barrier that appears suddenly. If the restriction is caused by edema, the sensation will be viscoelastic.

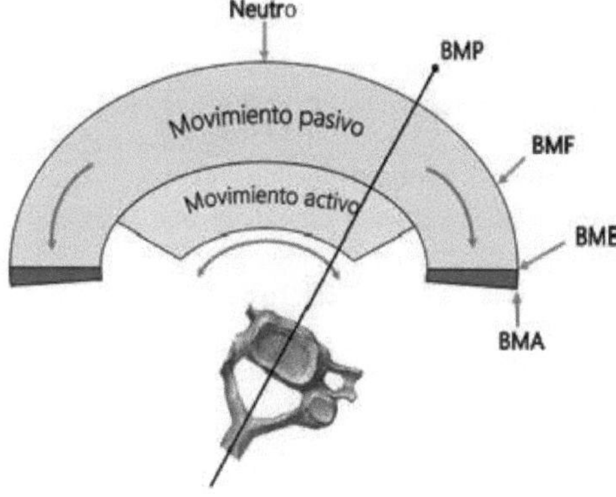

Figure 15. Barriers to joint movement (62).

On the other hand, Cyriax detailed the capsular restriction pattern of each joint, where the limitation of movement is caused by a restriction of the capsule, affecting certain movements more than others. It is important to consider that sometimes the limitation of movement does not have a mechanical origin, but a nociceptive origin (such as tendinopathies or nerve traction). In these cases, a sudden defensive muscle contraction may be perceived. Attention should also be paid to abnormal joint rhythms, which indicate asynchrony of movement. For example, in scapulohumeral rhythm, a prematurely moving scapula during abduction (before 60°) or an early lateral slip during shoulder external rotation suggest involvement of the shoulder joint capsule or a deficit in motor control. Finally, it is crucial to look for the presence of abnormal movements (such as knee recurvatum, elbow valgus, anterior or posterior knee drawer, etc.) that may indicate joint hyperlaxity. This hyperlaxity may be constitutional or suggestive of injury. To assess it, the Beighton scale is used, which considers the mobility of 5 joints and classifies a patient as hyperlax if he or she scores 4 or more out of a possible 9 points. Evaluation criteria include (63):

- Passive dorsiflexion of the 5th toe exceeding 90° (1 point per side).
- Thumbs passively reaching the flexor aspect of the forearm (1 point per side).
- Active hyperextension of the elbows reaching 10º (1 point per side).
- Hyperextension of the knees exceeding 10º (1 point per side).
- Forward flexion of the trunk with the knees in extension, so that the palms of the hands touch the floor (1 point).

Capsular pattern by joints according to Cyriax	
Articulation	**Capsular pattern**
Temporomandibular	Mouth opening
Cervical spine	Limited lateral tilt and rotation, full but painful flexion, limited extension.
Lumbar and thoracic spine	It is difficult to detect capsular pattern
Sacroiliac, pubic and sacroccygeal	Pain when stressing the joint.
Sternoclavicular and acromioclavicular	Pain in extreme ranges.

Shoulder	1º External rotation, 2º abduction and 3º internal rotation.
Elbow	More limited flexion than extension.
Distal radioulnar	Full ranges, but with pain at the end of the movement.
Doll	Equal limitation to flexion and extension, possible fixation in mid-position.
Thumb carpometacarpal	Full flexion, limitation in abduction and extension.
Phalanges	More limitation to flexion than to extension.
Hip	Internal rotation, flexion, abduction and extension.
Knee	Great limitation to flexion with slight limitation to extension. In early stages complete rotation and pain free.
Tibioperonea	Pain when stressing the joint.
Ankle	More limited plantar flexion than dorsal flexion.
Subastragaline	Limitation of investment.
Mediatarsal	Limitation of dorsal flexion, plantar flexion, adduction and internal rotation; abduction and external rotation retain full range.
Metatarsophalangeal of the first toe	More limited extension than flexion.
Metatarsophalangeal from second to fifth toe	Variable; tends to fixate in extension with flexion of the interphalangeal joints.

Table 9. Limitations in the capsular pattern by joints according to Cyriax (63).

In summary, manual assessment of joint mobility is a detailed and careful process that requires attention to multiple factors to correctly identify the causes of limitations or excesses in joint motion.

9.6. Joint proprioceptors

Self-perception refers to the body's ability to detect movement and joint position, which provides internal sensitivity. Cenesthesia is an integral part of self-perception and deals with awareness of movement and acceleration. Proprioceptors are important in controlling posture and balance, influencing coordination. Thus, the proprioceptive system is the source of somatic sensory information, composed of receptors that inform the central nervous system about the tension and stretch of muscles, joints, ligaments and skin, allowing necessary adjustments to achieve the desired movement. This process is rapid and subconscious, with the collaboration of vision and the vestibular system. Joint receptors are found in various joint structures (capsules, ligaments, etc.) and are mechanoreceptors. We can find: (64).

- Ruffini's corpuscles: Located in the outer layer of the joint capsule, ligaments and periosteum near the capsular insertions. Although they are distributed throughout the joint capsule, there are more in areas with greater mechanical stress. They are sensitive to low levels of stretching and have a slow adaptation, activating during prolonged joint stress and dynamic equilibrium, indicating the position, velocity and stress of the periarticular tissues (64).
  - Static: They record information in maintained positions.
  - Dynamic: They record information in continuous movements.
- Paccini's corpuscles: They are located in the external layer of the joint capsule, ligaments, menisci, joint fat and periosteum near the capsular insertions. They are mechanoreceptors of rapid adaptation, activating at the beginning and end of the movement to detect changes in tissue deformity and the acceleration or deceleration of joint movement (64).
- Free nerve endings: They are activated when joint movements exceed the normal range, causing painful sensations of alertness (64).

9.7. Instrumental joint assessment.

Quantitative measurement of joint mobility can be performed by several different methods. The following are detailed below:

9.7.1. Centimeter measurements:

To assess joint mobility, they are performed on different parts of the body and use different techniques specific to each area.

- Hand (65):
  - Digit-palm distance: The distance between the thumb of each long finger and the palm of the hand is measured in millimeters, evaluating the global flexion amplitude of the finger joints.
  - Distance between the thumb of each long finger and the flexion crease of the metacarpophalangeal joints: Measures the joint flexion amplitude of both interphalangeal joints.
  - Span measurement: The distance between the ends of the first and fifth fingers is measured with the hand open and the fingers at maximum separation.

- Distance between the ends of the first and second fingers at maximum separation: Measures the abduction of the thumb.

- Column (66):
  - Finger-floor distance: Evaluates the global mobility of the spine in anterior flexion, measuring the vertical distance between the thumb of the third finger and the floor with the knees in extension. It is non-specific and may indicate limited dorsolumbar mobility, ischiocrural shortening, presence of positive Lasègue or hip impairment.
  - Mandible-sternal manubrium distance: Assesses cervical flexion and extension.
  - Chin-acromion distance: For cervical rotations.
  - Acromion-atrial tragus distance: For cervical lateroflexion.
  - Measurement of dorsolumbar lateroflexion: With the patient standing and the hands on the outer thighs, a mark is drawn on the thigh at the level of the end of the third toe. Then mark again in right and left lateroflexion, and measure the distance between the marks.
  - Measurement of dorsolumbar rotation: The distance between the posterior edge of the acromion homolateral to the rotation and the contralateral posterosuperior superior iliac spine is measured.
  - Measurement of the movements and resting position of the scapula: Mobility in abduction-adduction and internal and external scales movements are assessed by measuring the distance from the inferior angle of the scapula to the D7 spinous process and from the internal border of the scapula spine to the D3 spinous process during movements. In normal position, the scapula lies between the 2nd and 7th ribs, with its superointernal angle at the level of the 1st dorsal spinous process, and the internal portion of the scapula spine at the level of the 3rd dorsal spinous process and 5-6 cm from the midline. The inferior angle of the scapula is located 7 cm from the midline at rest.
  - Ott test: It measures the flexibility of the dorsal spine by marking the spinous process of C7 and another mark 30 cm below. Flexion and extension of the spine are requested and the distance between

the two marks is measured in both positions. In flexion, the distance should increase by 2 to 4 cm, and in extension, it should decrease by 1 to 2 cm.

- Schöber test: It assesses the mobility of the lumbar spine by marking the spinous process of S1 and another mark 10 cm above. The distance variation in flexion and extension is measured. The standard is a distance of 15 cm in flexion and 9 cm in extension. MacRae and Wright's modification of the Schöber test includes three marks: one at the line joining the posterosuperior iliac spines, another 5 cm below and a third 10 cm above. The distance between the upper and lower marks is measured in flexion and maximal extension.

9.7.2. Goniometry

Goniometry is used to measure the angle of displacement of a bone segment in relation to the center of rotation of a joint. To do this, the center of the goniometer is placed in the cutaneous projection of the joint center. The fixed branch is directed towards a bony reference point at the proximal level and the mobile branch towards a bony reference point in the distal segment, ensuring that the goniometer is in the same plane as the movement and that its arms coincide with the longitudinal body axes (67).

- Principles to be followed (67):
  - Avoid compensations: Proximal joints are fixed.
  - Consider the muscular state: Pay attention to the tension or relaxation of the polyarticular muscles.
  - Initial evaluation of the healthy side: To have a reference.
  - Amplitudes on the dominant side: They are smaller on the upper limb than on the contralateral side.
  - Uncovered area to be evaluated: Important for an accurate measurement.
  - Consistency in the evaluation position: It is usually started at position zero and noted for future reevaluations.

- Bone landmarks: Alignment of the goniometer axis with the center of joint rotation (67).
  - Ankle: apex of the external malleolus.
  - Knee: 2.5 cm above the fibula head.

- Hip: Greater trochanter.
- Wrist: ulnar styloid for flexion-extension, center of interstyloid distance for abduction-adduction.
- Elbow: Epicondyle.
- Shoulder: Trochlea.

- Types of Goniometers (67).
    - Two-branch goniometers (universal or arthrometer): Conta of two arms attached to a common axis. The fixed arm is integrated with the body, which is an angle protractor in the form of a sphere graduated with 180º or 360º. The movable arm rotates around the axis and indicates the degrees.
    - Single-branch goniometers (orthocentric or plumb bob): A single arm that reads the angle formed with the plumb bob. Based on gravity, it must be in the vertical plane. Allows measurement of flexion-extension and abduction-adduction in standing position, as well as flexion-extension and rotations in different positions.
    - Electrogoniometer: Generates an electrical signal proportional to the joint displacement. It is more complex and precise.
    - Magnetic deflection goniometer (compass): Consists of a compass mounted on an arm. Used in the horizontal plane, with magnetic north as position 0. The cervical goniometer has a compass in each plane of space and a stabilizer.
    - Inclinometer: Ideal for areas where a conventional goniometer cannot be used (such as the lumbar spine). It uses gravity as a reference. It can be mechanical (with a liquid column and air bubble) or electronic (electroinclinometer).
    - Other types:
        - Finger and handlebar goniometers.
        - Spine measurement: spondylodoniometer and lumbo-pelvic-femoral rachiometer.
- Measurement Reading (67):
    - Angular values: Transcribed in 2 or 3 digit format with a margin of error of 5º. Grouped according to the plane of movement and according to the neutral position.
    - Direct reading: When the goniometer indicates 0º in neutral position, for example, elbow flexion-extension starts at 0º.

- Indirect reading: For joints whose reference position is not 0º. The initial value is subtracted from the angular if they are in the same sector of movement, and is added to the inverse sector.
- Special indications: If a joint does not reach the reference position, it must be indicated.

Movement		Grades
Upper extremity		
Shoulder	Abduction	180º
	Adduction	30º
	Flexion	180º
	Extension	50º
	Internal rotation	70º
	External rotation	90º
Elbow	Flexion	140-145º
	Extension	0º (5-10º)
Forearm	Pronation	85º
	Supination	90º
Doll	Flexion	85º
	Extension	85º
	Radial deviation	15-20º
	Ulnar deviation	30-45º
Lower extremity		
Hip	Flexion	120-145º
	Extension	30º
	Abduction	45º
	Adduction	30º
	Internal rotation	30-40º
	External rotation	60º
Knee	Flexion	160º
	Extension	0º (5-10º)
	Internal rotation (in flexion)	30º
	External rotation (in flexion)	40º
Ankle	Dorsal flexion	30º
	Plantar flexion	50º
Foot (subtalar)	Investment	30º
	Eversion	15º

Spine		
Cervical	Flexion (especially at C5-C6 level)	45º
	Extension (especially at C5-C6 level)	45º
	Lateral tilt	45º
	Rotation (especially at C1-C2 level)	80-90º
Dorsal	Ott's test: flexion-extension	2-4/1-2 cm
	Rotation	45º
	Thoracic expansion	6 cm
Lumbar	Flexion	40º-60º.
	Extension	30º
	Inclination	20-30º
	Rotation	15-20º

Table 10. Degrees of normal movement by joint (67).

9.8. Other measurements

9.8.1. Kaltenborn scale.

When instrumental assessment is not possible, the Kaltenborn Scale, which measures motion from 0 to 6, can be used, especially in joints with little motion (68):

0: Ankylosis
1: Significant limitation
2: Mild limitation
3: Normal
4: Slight increase in mobility
5: Significant increase in mobility
6: Joint instability

9.8.2. Kapandji Thumb Opposition Scale.

To assess the oppositional ability of the thumb, the Kapandji Scale, which ranges from 0 to 10, is used. The thumb can oppose the following points (65):

0: Lateral side of the first phalanx of the second finger.
1: Lateral side of the second phalanx of the second finger.

2: Lateral side of the third phalanx of the second finger.
3: Thumbnail of the second finger.
4: Thumbnail of the third finger.
5: Finger pad of the fourth finger.
6: Thumbnail of the fifth finger.
7: Distal interphalangeal joint of the fifth finger.
8: Proximal interphalangeal joint of the fifth finger.
9: Base of the fifth finger.
10: Flexion crease of the metacarpophalangeal joint of the fifth finger.

9.8.3. Kapandji's Three-Point Test.

Kapandji also describes a measurement of the global mobility of the shoulder joint complex. The test consists of marking the end of the third finger when the patient brings the hand to the back in the following positions (65):

- External flexion-rotation
- Extension-internal rotation
- Adduction over the contralateral shoulder

The surface of the triangle obtained gives an assessment of the mobility of the shoulder joint complex.

9.8.4. Star of Maigne.

To record the mobility of the spine, the Star of Maigne is used. It is a cross in which each of the upper sectors is crossed by a bisector (69):

- The upper segment represents bending.
- The lower one represents the extension.
- The left and right arms represent the rotations.
- The left and right bisectors represent the lateral inclinations.

In each segment the limitation of movement is indicated (near the center if it is at the beginning of the physiological amplitude and towards the end if it is at the end) and its cause:

- With a cross if it is for a blockage.
- With one, two or three bars if it is for mild, moderate or severe pain.

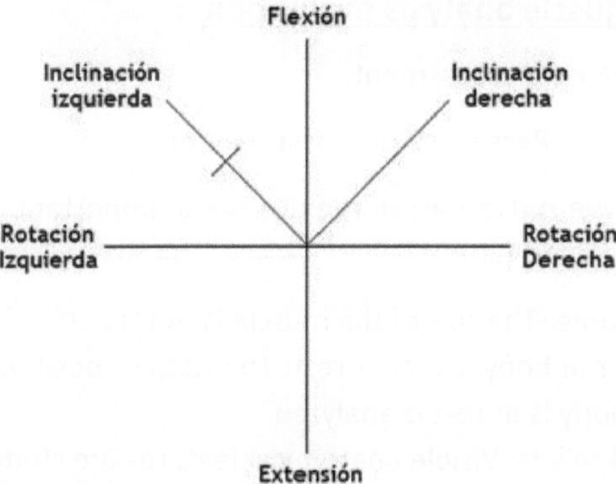

Figure 16. Star of Maigne. A joint block is indicated for left tilt (69).

10. Muscle analysis evaluation

10.1. Muscle assessment.

10.1.1. Passive muscle assessment.

In passive muscle assessment, several important aspects of the muscle are observed (70):

- Muscle volume: The size of the muscle is examined.
- Position of the bony levers at rest: The natural position of the bones when the body is at rest is analyzed.
- Anatomical reliefs: Visible anatomical features are studied.
- Base Muscle Tone: The state of tension of the muscle at absolute rest, without any contraction, including antigravity, is evaluated.

If the state of tension of the muscle during an action against gravity is assessed, it is referred to as postural tone. To assess muscle tone, the following are considered (70):

- Modifications in body posture
- Osteotendinous reflexes
- Ability to execute the movement freely
- Resistance to passive mobilization
- Palpation and Tissue Mobilization: They provide information on muscle consistency and transverse passive mobility. In very weak muscles, palpation can detect muscle activity.
- Tendon: It does not change its consistency during muscle contraction, but its transverse mobility decreases proportionally to the force generated.
- Extensibility: It is assessed by placing the muscle in a position of maximum stretch at each joint it crosses. If the muscle does not fully elongate, a partial loss of movement called retraction is detected.
- Muscular Insufficiency:
    - Passive Functional: When a muscle is stretched to its maximum and cannot be stretched any further.
    - Functional Active: When the muscle is at maximum shortening and can no longer contract due to maximum overlapping of actin and myosin filaments.

- Myofascial Trigger Points (MTrPs): Hyperirritable areas within a tight band of skeletal muscle that cause local and referred pain and motor dysfunction.

10.1.2. Active muscle assessment.

For the evaluation of active contraction, the maximum resistance that a muscle can overcome is quantified by calculating the static and dynamic RM (repetition maximum) and the 10RM using external loads (70).

- Factors to Consider (70):
  - Anatomical, biomechanical and physiological knowledge.
  - Cancellation of substitution movements (Beevor's axiom).
  - Proper positioning of the segment to be assessed, starting in an antigravitational position.
  - Skill in palpation and application of external resistance.
  - Clear explanation to the patient.
  - Use of a standardized method of force grading.
  - Experience in muscle balancing.
  - Place and direction of application of the resistance.
- Qualitative Assessment: Strength can be assessed qualitatively according to the ability of a muscle to overcome gravity, known as muscle balance. The patient is not symmetrical, so the musculature on one side may be stronger than the other, but it is assessed by comparison with the healthy side.

10.1.3. Scales for the evaluation of muscle strength.

Strength grading scales are essential tools in physical therapy to assess the contractile capacity of muscles. These scales allow muscle strength to be measured qualitatively and quantitatively, providing a systematic guide to identify the level of muscle function and detect possible weaknesses or imbalances. Muscle strength assessments are crucial both in diagnosing injuries and in monitoring rehabilitation progress and planning muscle strengthening programs. Different scales, such as the Oxford scale, provide a standardized framework that facilitates comparison and communication of results between health professionals (70).

Scales for muscle strength assessment

Lowett (1912)	bad, poor, weak, good and normal	
Kendall (1946)	100% (normal)	Full movement against gravity and maximum resistance.
	75% (good)	Full movement against gravity and moderate resistance.
	50% (regular)	Complete movement against gravity without resistance.
	25% (bad)	Complete motion without the force of gravity.
	10% (vestiges)	Muscle contraction without movement.
	0%	Absence of muscle contraction.
Pinzler	0	No movement.
	+	Start of the movement.
	++	Incomplete movement.
	+++	Complete movement.
Daniels, Williams and Worthingham (Oxford Scale)	Grade 0 (0%)	Total absence of contractility.
	Grade 1 (10%)	Visible or palpable muscle contraction without movement.
	Grade 2 (25%)	Full motion eliminating gravity.
	Grade 3 (50%)	Complete movement against gravity.
	Grade 4 (75%)	Full movement against gravity and moderate resistance.
	Grade 5 (100%)	Full movement against maximum resistance.

Table 11. Scales for muscle assessment (70).

- Breaking and Active Resistance Test (70):
    - Rupture test: Apply manual resistance and ask the patient to maintain the position.
    - Active resistance test: Apply resistance opposite to muscular contraction until the maximum tolerated level is reached.

- Final Considerations: Manual muscle testing is reliable for detecting severe weakness, but shows variability at high forces. Muscle balance is useful for peripheral neurological and spinal cord injuries, but not for injuries of encephalic origin, where a more global and functional evaluation is required (70).

10.1.4. Instrumental measures for muscle assessment.

- Tape measure: The tape measure is used to measure changes in muscle volume during contraction and relaxation phases. This tool provides data on muscle size and can help monitor a patient's progress during rehabilitation or training (70).
- Dynamometers: Dynamometers are instruments designed to measure the isometric force that a muscle can generate. By assessing isometric force, an accurate measure of the muscle's ability to generate tension without changing its length is obtained (70).
- Isokinetic machine: Isokinetic machines allow concentric (when the muscle is shortened) and eccentric (when the muscle is lengthened) muscle contractions at a constant speed throughout the entire range of joint movement. These machines offer the advantage of adjusting the speed of the movement, which allows the activation of different types of muscle fibers according to the selected speed. This is useful for precise rehabilitation and for optimizing sports performance (70).

11. Functional assessment in physiotherapy

11.1. Examination of statics.

11.1.1. Observation.

Observation is an essential part of the assessment, as it provides a comprehensive view of the patient in his or her most natural state, complementing the information obtained from more structured and specific assessments. The concept of "normality" in terms of posture is complex due to the diversity among individuals and the variability that may depend on factors such as age, pathologies, fatigue state, among others. Even the same individual may show postural variations at different times of his or her life. This concept is closely linked to the morphotype of each person. Characteristics that should be present in a correctly aligned posture (71):

- Horizontal gaze: The head should be in such a position that the gaze is directed horizontally.
- Sagittal alignment: Occiput, mid-dorsal region and sacrum. These points should be aligned in the sagittal plane.
- Physiological sagittal curvatures:
  - Cervical and lumbar lordosis: Inward curvatures in the cervical and lumbar regions.
  - Dorsal kyphosis: outward curvature in the dorsal region.
- Alignment of the shoulder girdle and shoulders: The shoulders and shoulder girdle should be aligned horizontally.
- Alignment of the iliac bones: The iliac bones should also be aligned in the transverse axis.
- Unrolled shoulders: There should be absence of vertical or transverse rolling of the scapula.
- Neutral pelvis: Intermediate position of the pelvic scale. The pelvis should be in a neutral position, neither tilted forward (anteversion) nor backward (retroversion).
- Alignment of EIAS and pubic symphysis: The right and left anterior superior iliac spines (EIAS) should be aligned with the pubic symphysis in the same plane.
- Knees aligned in extension 0º: Knees should be aligned without flexion, recurvatum (hyperextension), varus (bowed) or valgus (knock-kneed).
- Calcaneus without varus or valgus: The heels should be aligned without inward (varus) or outward (valgus) tilt.

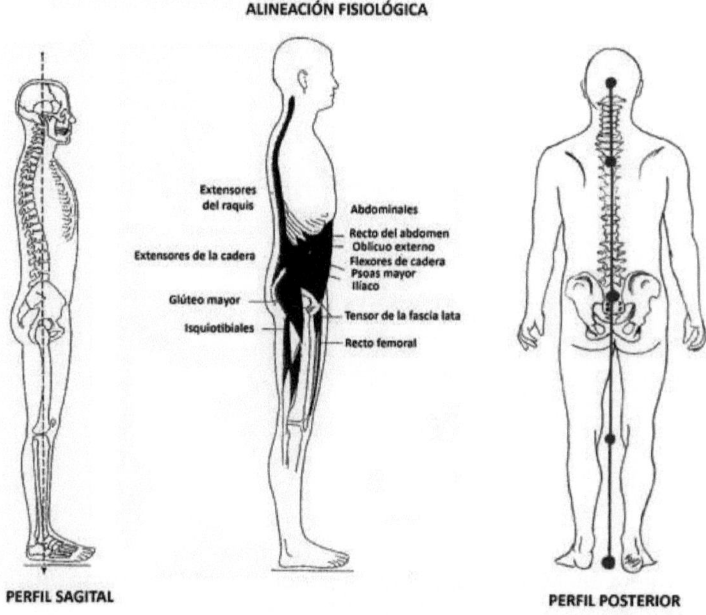

Figure 17. Ideal physiological alignment (9).

The following is a description of the different types of typical postures that can be observed, together with their characteristics and possible clinical implications (71):

- Superior Cruciate (or Shoulder) Syndrome:
  - Characteristics: Elevation and protraction of the shoulders, rotation and abduction of the scapulae, anteriorized head.
  - Implications: This syndrome can lead to problems such as neck pain, headaches and shoulder girdle dysfunction.

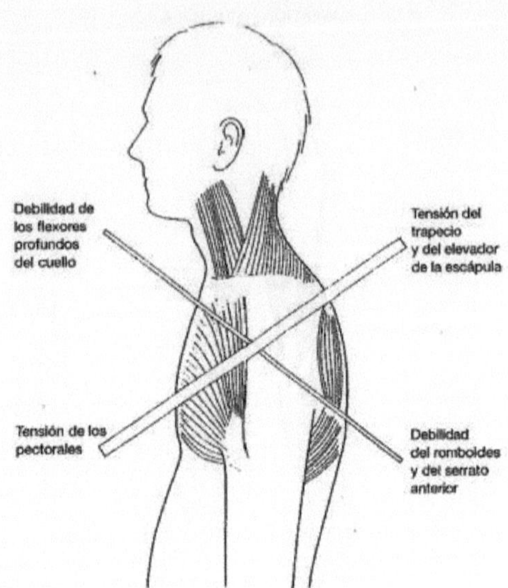

Figure 18. Morphology of the superior cruciate syndrome (9).

- Kyphosis-Lordosis posture (71):
    - Characteristics: Combination of lumbar hyperlordosis and thoracic hyperkyphosis, similar to upper and lower crossed syndromes.
    - Implications: This posture can cause generalized back pain and respiratory problems due to the alteration of the rib cage.

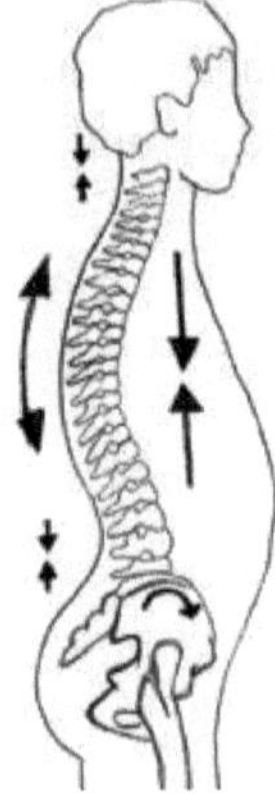

Figure 19. Posture in kyphosis-lordosis (9).

- Inferior cruciate (or pelvic) syndrome (71):

- Characteristics: Pelvic anteversion, increased lumbar lordosis, semi-flexion of the hips.
- Implications: This pattern may be associated with low back pain, hip problems and trunk stabilizing muscle dysfunction.

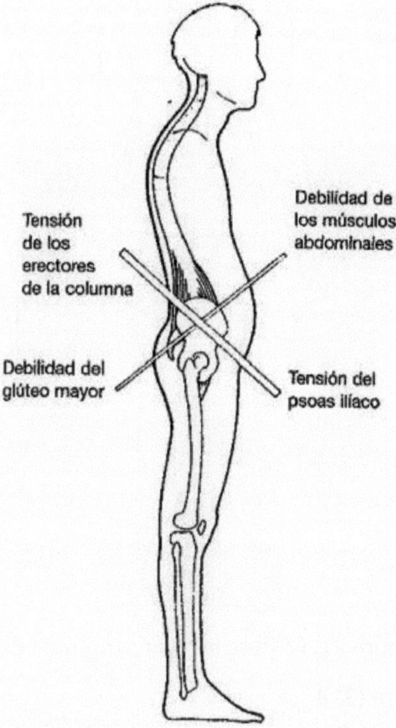

Figure 20. Morphology of the inferior cruciate syndrome (9).

- Layers Syndrome (71):
  - Characteristics: Alternating hypertrophic and hypotrophic muscles; weakness of scapula stabilizers, lumbosacral erectors, gluteus maximus, and abdominal muscles.
  - Implications: May lead to chronic back pain, pelvic instability and global postural problems.

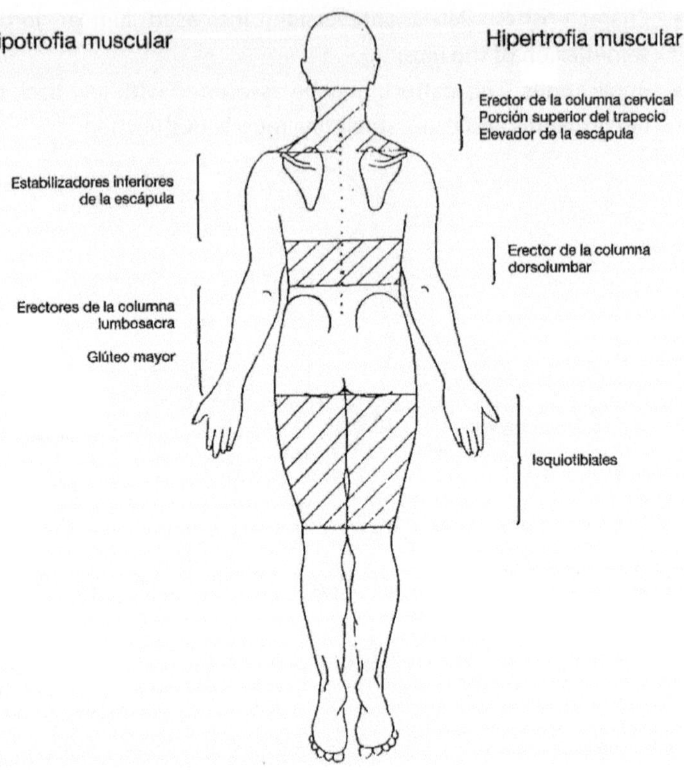

Figure 21. Posture in layer syndrome (9).

- Flat Back Posture (71):
    - Characteristics: Cervical spine slightly extended, upper part of the dorsal spine flexed, absence of lumbar lordosis, posterior tilt of the pelvis, extension of the hips.
    - Implications: This posture can result from weak, elongated hip flexors and shortened, strong hamstrings, contributing to low back pain and gait dysfunction.

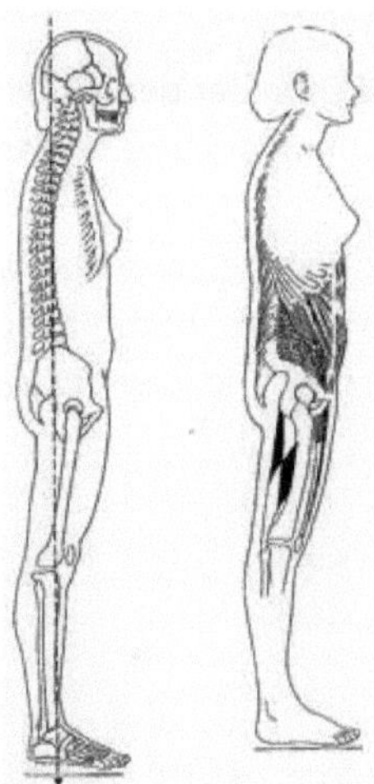

Figure 22. Flat back posture (9).

- Oscillating Back Posture (71):
    - Characteristics: anteriorized head, cervical spine extended, flexion and posterior displacement of the trunk, posterior tilting of the pelvis, hyperextended hips.
    - Implications: Related to elongation and weakness of hip flexors and abdominal muscles, and hamstring shortening, causing postural instability and low back pain.

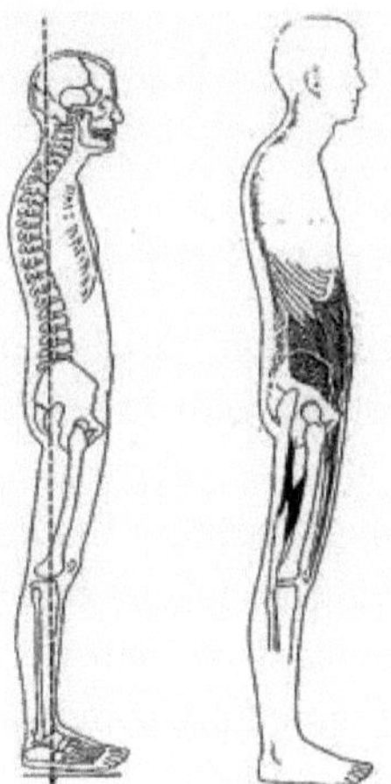

Figure 23. Oscillating back posture (9).

- Lateralized Posture (71):
  - Characteristics: Right shoulder descended, right scapula in descent and adduction, dorsolumbar curve convex to the left, lateral pelvic tilt.
  - Implications: May originate muscular imbalances between the right and left sides of the body, affecting the symmetry and functionality of the trunk and lower extremities.

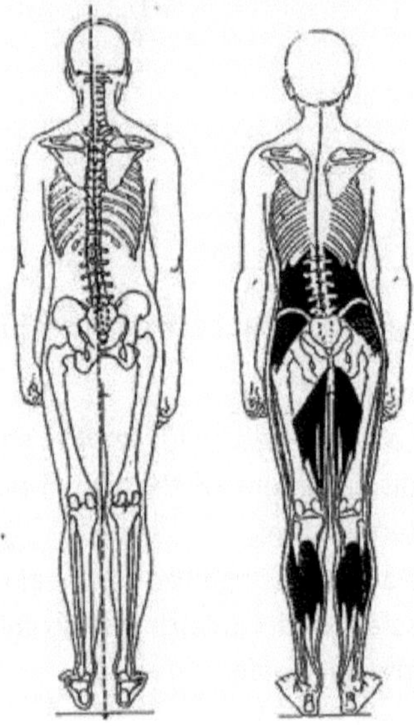

Figure 24. Lateralized posture (9).

11.2. Evaluation of normal gait

Human gait is the usual form of locomotion of man, allowing movement in bipedal position with low effort and minimum energy expenditure. This process involves alternating and rhythmic movements of the limbs and trunk, which facilitate the advancement of the body's center of gravity. The basic functional unit of gait is the gait cycle or stride, which comprises the sequence of movements between two consecutive contacts of the heel of the same foot, comprising two steps (72, 73).

During each gait cycle, each leg goes through two phases (72, 73):

- Support or stance phase: The leg is in contact with the ground, starting with heel contact and ending with forefoot toe-off. This phase includes two periods of double support (both feet on the ground) and two periods of monopodal support (one foot on the ground). It constitutes approximately 60% of the cycle.
- Swing phase: The leg comes off the ground and moves forward for the next support. It begins with the take-off of the forefoot and ends with the next contact of the foot with the ground, constituting the remaining 40% of the cycle.

Gait is characterized by the constant contact of at least one foot with the ground. At higher speeds, the bipodal support phase decreases and may disappear, marking the transition to running, where there are no bipodal supports and periods of monopodal support alternate with moments when both feet are in the air (72, 73).

The basic functional unit of walking is the gait cycle. This cycle is defined as the sequence of events that occur between two consecutive heel contacts of the same foot. Therefore, a long stride includes two steps, comprising from the support of one heel to the support of the opposite heel. The gait consists of the following features (72, 73):

- Stride length: Distance between two successive supports of the same heel.
- Step length: Distance between the support of one heel and that of the other heel.
- Pitch width: Distance between the midpoints of both heels in support.
- Pitch angle: Angle between the longitudinal axis of the foot and the line of march.
- Walking cadence: Number of steps per minute.
- Walking speed: Distance traveled in a unit of time. It is the product of the stride length and the walking cadence.

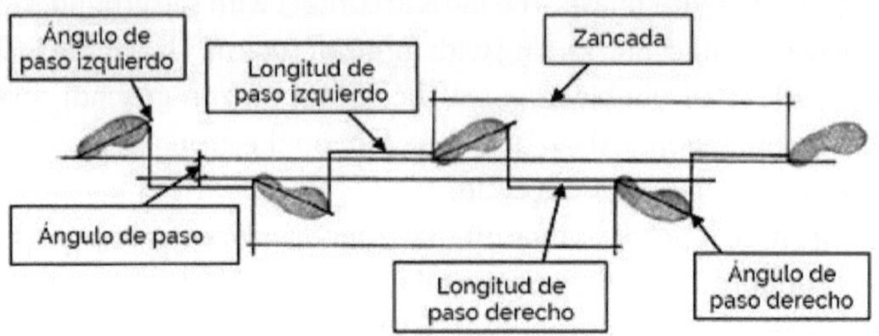

Figure 25. Gait parameters (73).

- Morphological Description of the Gait (74):

For gait analysis, the right foot is usually taken as the reference. The cycle starts with the first double stance (also known as the anterior stance phase of receiving and braking), which spans from the contact of the right heel with the ground to the toe-off of the left foot. This phase starts at 0% of the cycle and ends around 10%. Then, between 10% and 50% of the cycle, the right lower limb monopodal stance (MID) phase develops. This phase begins with the toe-off of the left foot (specifically the first toe) and ends with the heel of the same foot resting on the ground, so that the MID is in contact with the ground while the left foot performs its swing period. Between 50% and 60% of the cycle, the second phase of bipodal stance (also called posterior impulsion stance) takes place, which comprises from the left heel landing to the toe-off of the right foot. The cycle continues with the oscillation of the MID during monopodal stance on the left lower extremity, from toe-off of the right toe to the new stance of the right heel, which corresponds to 100% of the cycle. These divisions of the gait cycle can be subdivided into smaller phases, such as those proposed by Perry in 1992.

The gait cycle is analyzed using the right foot as a reference and is divided into stance and swing phases (74).

- Phase 1. Support phase (74):
  - Initial contact (0-2% of the cycle):
    - The right foot touches the ground with the edge of the heel.
    - The knee is almost extended, the hip flexed at 30° and the right pelvis forward.
    - Active muscles:

- Erectors of the spine: Manage the flexion and inclination of the torso.
- Gluteus maximus: Activate at the end of the swing to drive the hip during initial contact and begin extension when loading weight.
- Gluteus medius: Active in the final swing phase and throughout the stance phase, it stabilizes the pelvis with eccentric isotonic contraction, preventing its lateral oscillation. Other muscles such as the gluteus minimus, tensor fascia lata and the contralateral quadratus lumborum help in this stabilization.
- Adductor magnus: Works at the end of the swing along with the gluteus medius to maintain pelvic balance.
- Quadriceps: Contracts concentrically at the end of the swing to extend the knee before heel contact and control the flexion caused by the hamstrings.
- Hamstrings: Collaborate with the quadriceps, contracting eccentrically at the end of the swing to control knee extension and then concentrically to flex the knee after heel contact.

- Response to load (2-10% of the cycle):
  - The right foot makes full contact with the ground.
  - Active muscles:
    - Gluteus maximus: They perform hip extension.
    - Gluteus medius, gluteus medius minimus and tensor fascia lata: stabilize the pelvis in the frontal plane, and the tensor fascia lata also ensures lateral stability of the knee.
    - Quadriceps: modulates knee flexion eccentrically.
    - Peroneus longus and posterior tibialis: activated at the end of the phase to control ankle movements in the lateral plane during monopodal stance.
- Medium support (10-30% of the cycle):
  - The left foot takes off and the right foot supports the weight of the body.
  - Active muscles:
    - Gluteus maximus: it contracts concentrically at the beginning of the monopodal support, stopping when reaching the vertical position.

- Gluteus medius, gluteus medius, gluteus minimus and tensor fascia lata: keep the pelvis stable in the lateral plane.
- Quadriceps: contracts concentrically to extend the knee at the beginning of the phase.
- Hamstrings: regulate knee extension at the beginning and, together with the quadriceps, cease their activity at the end of the phase.
- Triceps suralis (mainly soleus): controls the anterior movement of the tibia over the ankle eccentrically.
- Posterior tibial and peroneal: ensure foot stability.

- Final support (30-50% of the cycle):
  - The tibia passes from vertical, the ankle flexes dorsally, and the knee and hip extend.
  - Active muscles: psoas iliacus, gluteus medius and gluteus minimus, tensor fascia latae, triceps suralis, tibialis posterior, peroneus, and flexor digitorum longus.
    - Psoas iliacus: contracts eccentrically to stop hip extension.
    - Gluteus medius, gluteus minimus and tensor fascia lata: remain active to stabilize the pelvis laterally, ceasing at the end of the phase.
    - Triceps suralis: it contracts concentrically with force for heel take-off and acceleration of the body.
    - Posterior tibial and lateral peroneals: remain active.
    - Flexor digitorum longus and first toe: contract concentrically during heel strike.
- Pre-oscillation (50-60% of the cycle):
  - The right foot prepares to take off while the left heel touches the ground.
  - Active muscles:
    - Spinal erectors: manage the anterior torso tilt after left heel contact.
    - Hip flexors (psoas): contract concentrically to propel the leg forward.
    - Quadriceps (rectus femoris): contracts eccentrically to prevent knee flexion caused by the triceps suralis and assists the psoas in hip flexion.

- Triceps suralis and tibialis posterior: they contract concentrically to perform plantar flexion of the ankle and push the foot forward.
- Peroneus lateralis longus: concentrically controls the supinator action of the tibialis posterior during plantar flexion of the ankle.

- Phase 2. Oscillation phase (74):
  - Initial oscillation (60-73% of the cycle):
    - The right foot lifts off the ground and the limb is shortened to avoid hitting the ground.
    - Active muscles:
      - Psoas-iliac and adductor magnus: contract concentrically to flex the hip, shortening the limb and propelling it forward.
      - Quadriceps (rectus femoris): contracts eccentrically to control knee flexion and assists in hip flexion.
      - Hamstrings: contract concentrically to flex the knee.
      - Anterior tibialis, common extensor of the toes and extensor of the first toe: they perform dorsal flexion to prevent the foot from stumbling on the ground.
  - Medium oscillation (73-87% of the cycle):
    - The right foot advances, the knee begins to passively extend and the ankle reaches a neutral position.
    - Active muscles:
      - Psoas-iliac: only active at the beginning of the phase.
      - Hamstrings: start an eccentric contraction to slow the acceleration of the limb forward.
      - Anterior tibialis, common extensor of the fingers and extensor of the first finger.
  - Final oscillation (87-100% of the cycle):
    - The right foot prepares for ground contact, the knee is extended and the ankle is in neutral position.
    - Active muscles:
      - Gluteus maximus, gluteus medius and gluteus minimus: contract to prepare for new heel contact.
      - Quadriceps: extend the knee for initial contact with the heel.
      - Hamstrings and popliteus: they contract eccentrically to stop knee extension, with maximum activation in this phase.

- Anterior tibialis, common extensor of the toes and extensor of the first toe: continue to be active concentrically to prepare the heel for ground contact.

This detailed description of human gait is essential for biomechanical analysis and diagnosis of gait pattern alterations, which in turn helps in the planning of appropriate therapeutic interventions. Below is a summary table of the different stages of gait.

PHASES OF THE GAIT CYCLE			
Support phase			
Initial contact	**Gait cycle**	0-2% of cycle	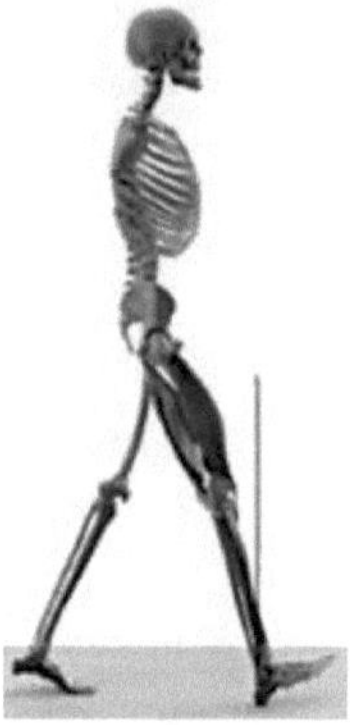
	Hip	30°	
	Knee	0-5°	
	Ankle	0°	
	Muscle activity	Erectors of the spine, gluteus maximus, gluteus medius, adductor magnus, quadriceps, hamstrings	
	Function	Heel contact with the ground	
Initial support. Response to load	**Gait cycle**	2-10% of the cycle	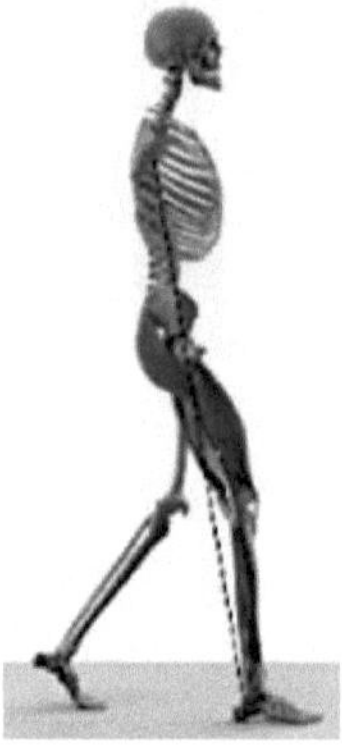
	Hip	30°	
	Knee	20°	
	Ankle	5-10° plantar flexion	
	Muscle activity	Gluteus maximus, gluteus medius and minimus, tensor fascia lata, quadriceps, peroneus longus lateralis and tibialis posterior.	
	Function	Knee and ankle shock absorption. Load transfer and hip stability. Forward movement by heel roll.	
Medium support	**Gait cycle**	10-30%	

	Hip	10°	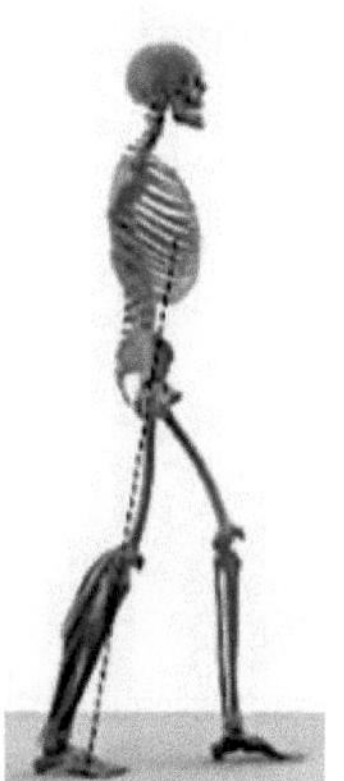
	Knee	0-5°	
	Ankle	5° dorsal flexion	
	Muscle activity	Gluteus maximus, medius and minimus, tensor fascia lata, quadriceps, hamstrings, triceps suralis, tibialis posterior and peroneals.	
	Function	Forward movement by controlling the tibia. Moving the center of gravity forward by rocking the ankle.	
Final support	Gait cycle	30-50%	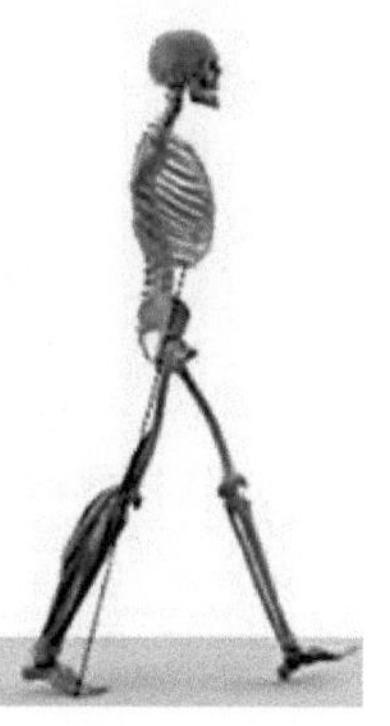
	Hip	10° hyperextension	
	Knee	0-5° flexion	
	Ankle	10° plantar flexion 30° extension of the metatarsophalangeal joints	
	Muscle activity	Psoas iliacus, gluteus medius and gluteus minimus, tensor fascia lata, triceps suralis, tibialis posterior, peroneus, and flexor digitorum longus.	
	Function	The second roller generates forward motion, moving the center of gravity away from the support base and ensuring proper stride length. Controlled plantar flexion of the ankle, lifting the heel off the ground.	

Pre-oscillation	Gait cycle	50-60% 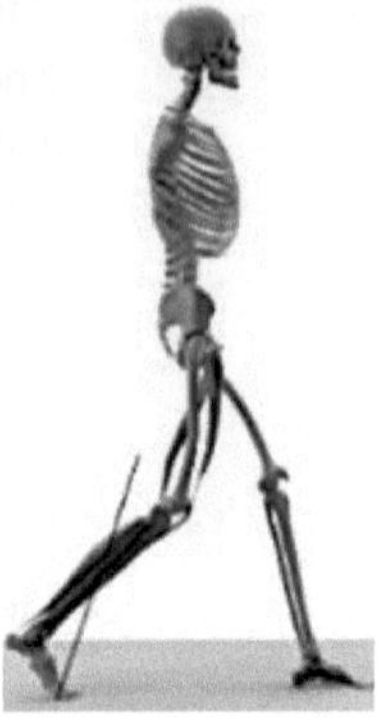
	Hip	-10° hyperextension
	Knee	40° flexion
	Ankle	15° plantar flexion
	Muscle activity	spinal erectors, hip flexors (psoas), quadriceps, triceps suralis, posterior tibialis, and peroneus longus lateralis.
	Function	Passive knee flexion of 40°. Plantar flexion of the ankle.
Oscillation phase		
Initial oscillation	Gait cycle	60-73% 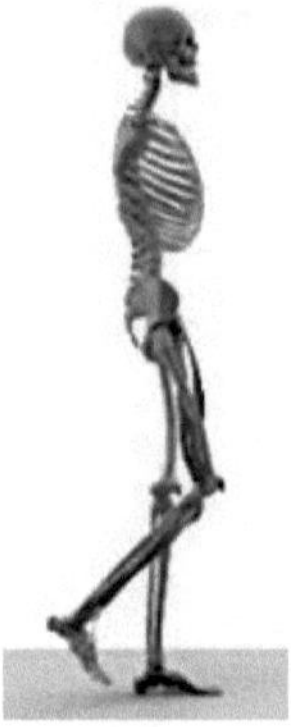
	Hip	15° flexion
	Knee	60-70° flexion
	Ankle	5° plantar flexion
	Muscle activity	psoas-iliac, adductor magnus, quadriceps, hamstrings, and dorsal flexors.
	Function	Knee flexion of at least 55° for sufficient ground clearance.
Average oscillation	Gait cycle	73-87% 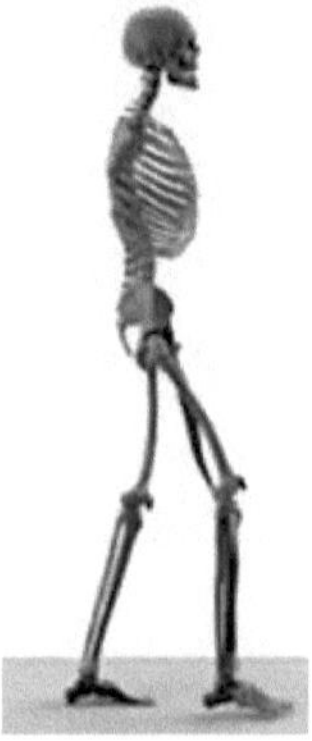
	Hip	25° flexion
	Knee	25° flexion
	Ankle	0°
	Muscle activity	Psoas-iliac (initially), hamstrings (eccentrically), and dorsal flexors.
	Function	Increasing hip flexion to 25°, ankle movement to neutral position.

Final oscillation	Gait cycle	87-100%
	Hip	20° flexion
	Knee	0-5° flexion
	Ankle	0°
	Muscle activity	Gluteus maximus, gluteus medius and gluteus minimus
	Function	Knee extension to neutral flexion and preparation for stance phase.

Table 12. Summary of the complete gait cycle with the different phases (74).

- Behavior of the pelvis, trunk and upper limbs during gait: During gait, the pelvis, trunk and upper limbs execute coordinated movements in the three planes of space (74).
    - Pelvis: In the frontal plane, the pelvis remains in an anteversion of 10-12° during almost the entire cycle, with variations of 4° towards retroversion in monopodal support. With respect to the frontal plane it performs upward and downward movements with an amplitude of approximately 5°. It is horizontal at initial contact, rises at the end of the initial stance phase, and descends during pre-swing and initial swing, controlled by the hip abductors. In the transverse plane the pelvis is rotated internally during initial contact and externally during preoscillation.
    - Trunk: Performs rotation, inclination and lateral oscillation movements. There is an opposite movement between the pelvic and shoulder girdle, with the shoulder forward in the initial contact and delayed in the preoscillation.
    - Upper limbs: They perform flexion and extension movements of 45-50°. The movements are synchronized and opposed homolaterally, that is, while an upper limb moves forward, the lower limb on the same side moves backward. The elbow follows a flexion-extension pattern similar to that of the shoulder, although with a slight delay.

This set of movements ensures the coordination and balance necessary for efficient walking (74).

- Displacement of the center of gravity and energy-saving factors during gait: The center of gravity of the body is located near the second sacral vertebra, at approximately 55% of the height of the person from the ground. During gait, this center does not follow a straight line, but forms a double sinusoidal curve in the cranio-caudal and latero-medial directions, with an amplitude of 5 cm and 4 cm respectively. The highest point of the curve is located in the middle phase of the monopodal stance, while the lowest point is located in the double stance phase. To reduce energy consumption and make gait more efficient, there are six mechanisms that decrease the amplitude of the center of gravity shifts, known as "gait determinants" or "gait optimization mechanisms":
  - Pelvis rotation in the transverse plane: The pelvis rotates about 4° during hip flexion-extension, lengthening the gait without increasing the vertical displacement of the center of gravity.
  - Pelvic tilt in the frontal plane: The pelvis tilts about 5° towards the swinging side during monopodal support, reducing the upward displacement of the center of gravity.
  - Knee flexion in stance phase: The knee flexes about 15° after initial heel contact, decreasing the vertical oscillation of the center of gravity.
  - Coordination of ankle and knee movements: The synchronization of these movements avoids deceleration and abrupt start of the center of gravity at the beginning and end of the support.
  - Foot and ankle movements: Plantar flexion of the ankle at heel contact and dorsal flexion at take-off allow a smoother displacement of the center of gravity.
  - Lateral displacement of the pelvis: The pelvis shifts laterally to align the center of gravity with the heel of support, reducing the base of support and lateral displacements.

In addition, it has been proposed that upper limb braking should be considered a determinant of gait, as it helps to reduce energy expenditure and vertical displacement of the center of gravity during gait.

11.3. Scales for gait evaluation

Gait study is essential for diagnosing neurological and musculoskeletal diseases and evaluating patient interventions. Gait can be assessed by:

- Observational assessment: Direct observation or recordings allow the identification of alterations in movement patterns.
- Standardized scales:
  - Rivermead Visual Gait Assessment (RVGA): Includes 20 items that assess lower limbs, trunk and upper limbs, with scores from 0 (normal) to 3 (severe impairment) (75).
  - Wisconsin Gait Scale (WGS): Consists of 13 items that assess the lower limb in different phases of gait and one item for the use of support products (76).
  - Gait Assessment and Intervention Tool (GAIT): Contains 31 items that assess lower limbs, upper limbs and trunk in stance and swing phases, with different ordinal scales (77).
  - Tinetti Gait Scale (TGS): Assesses gait and balance (78).
  - Gait Abnormality Rating Scale (GARS): Designed to assess gait abnormalities in geriatric patients (79).
- Instrumental evaluation (80):
  - Electrogoniometers: They measure joint amplitude both at rest and dynamically.
  - Accelerometers: Measure the orientation, position and acceleration of an object.
  - Photogrammetry and videogrammetry systems: They use markers and cameras to digitally reconstruct the movement in a three-dimensional manner.
  - Dynamometry platforms: They measure the forces exerted against the ground and the ground reaction force.
  - Dynamic electromyography: Analyzes muscle activation and effort intensity during walking.
  - Electronic podoscopes: Devices placed in the footwear that provide information on the distribution of plantar pressures during gait.

11.4. Evaluation of pathological gait

The gait pattern is specific to each individual and is influenced by intrinsic (age, sex, etc.), extrinsic (terrain, footwear, load carried, etc.), psychological and pathological (neurological, musculoskeletal, etc.) factors that can cause temporary or permanent alterations. The causes of pathological gait are pain, musculoskeletal abnormalities, neurological lesions (central and peripheral).

There are different types of pathological gait (73, 74, 81):

- Steppage gait (also known as equinus, drop foot, tabetic or soldier's gait): Support is provided by the toe or sole of the foot. It is characterized by a foot tapping at the beginning due to a drop of the forefoot in the swing phase and an exaggerated flexion of the hip and knee to prevent the toe from touching the ground, due to the loss of dorsiflexion of the ankle due to weakness of the dorsiflexor musculature of the foot. This gait occurs in patients with L5 radiculopathy, sciatic or deep peroneal neuropathy and polyneuropathies (alcoholism, vitamin B12 deficiency and diabetes).
- Hemiparetic or reaper's gait (scything): Hemiparetic or reaper's gait, also known as scything, results from unilateral lesion of the corticospinal pathway or motor cortex. It is characterized by a hip circumduction movement due to increased tone in knee extension and plantar flexion of the ankle. This gait is observed in patients with hemiplegia or paresis of the lower extremity. Throughout the gait cycle, the affected lower extremity remains extended. Two main problems can be identified:
    - In the stance phase, when transferring weight, a proper balance reaction does not occur, resulting in an elevation of the center of gravity and a dropping of the pelvis to the opposite side due to lack of strength in the abductor muscles.
    - During the swing phase, the leg performs a circular motion and the pelvis rises to compensate for the movement. To counteract this compensation, it is necessary to flex the knee with the hip extended, keeping the pelvis in position, and then bring the flexed knee forward with dorsal flexion of the foot, thus describing a cone-shaped movement.

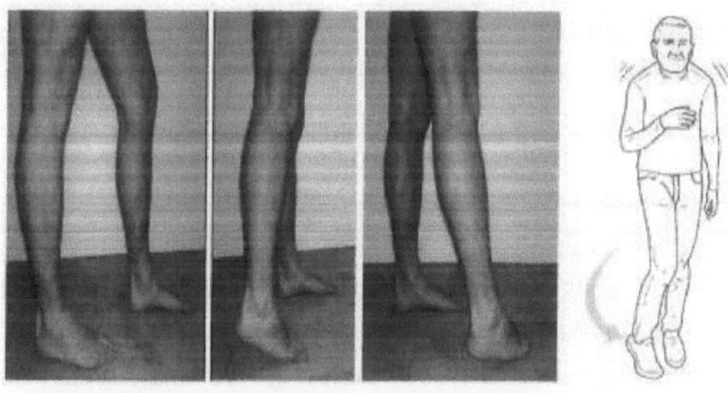

Figure 26. Hemiparetic or reaper gait pattern (74).

- Festatory (propulsive, hasty, parkinsonian) gait: Parkinson's disease is a chronic, progressive, irreversible degenerative condition that affects the brain's dopaminergic pathways. It is the second most common neurodegenerative disease after Alzheimer's disease. It has no definitive clinical marker for diagnosis. The most characteristic lesions in Parkinson's disease are depigmentation of the substantia nigra and locus coeruleus due to loss of neurons. Lewy bodies, rounded cytoplasmic inclusions, are observed in the remaining neurons. The main biochemical problem in Parkinson's disease is the reduction of dopamine in the substantia nigra and striatum, which hinders the execution of movements and causes rigidity. This is due to a decrease in the enzymes that synthesize dopamine while those that degrade it remain normal, resulting in an imbalance between dopamine and acetylcholine.

James Parkinson described in 1817 the postural and gait disorders in this disease: flexion of the chin to the chest, trunk leaning forward, short and rapid steps, and the transition from a normal gait to a near-running gait. It is now recognized that the typical posture of Parkinson's patients is with flexion of the trunk and limbs, and a narrow base of support. Gait is usually normal in the early stages of the disease; an early and severe gait disturbance suggests other possible diagnoses. Gait problems and postural instability in Parkinson's have multifactorial causes, related to altered righting reflexes, rigidity and akinesia. Symptoms such as akinesia, hypokinesia, bradykinesia, difficulty in simultaneous and sequential movements, and hypersensitivity to external stimuli that cause motor blocks, affect mobility and independence in daily activities, impairing quality of life.

- Characteristics of Parkinson's Gait
  - Upper limbs: Decreased brachiation, one of the first signs of the disease.
  - Lower limbs: Temporal and spatial variability in the regularity and stability of gait, with short steps, little elevation of the feet and decreased speed.
  - Freezing: Difficulty in initiating walking, which is often associated with turns and can lead to falls.
  - Festination: Short, rapid steps, especially when attempting to perform another task simultaneously.
  - Arrhythmokinesis: Inability to maintain a constant rhythm in repetitive movements, considered a predictive factor for falls.

Correct identification and assessment of altered gait patterns are essential to improve locomotor pattern symmetry and patient independence. Gait assessment scales include the Modified Parkinson Activity Scale (M-PAS), Timed Up and Go (TUG), Mini-BESTest, and others.

Parkinson's patients experience more falls than the general population of the same age. These falls are related to disease progression, drug treatment complications and aging. A clinical evaluation complemented by the administration of scales is essential to improve the therapeutic management of these patients.

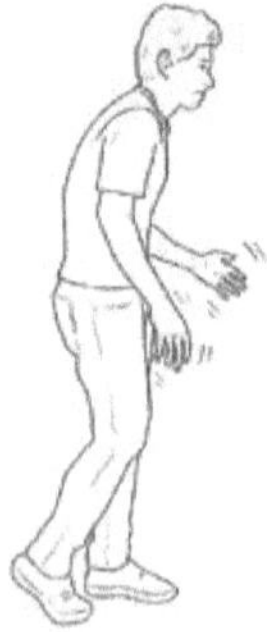

Figure 27. Festinant gait pattern (74).

- Trendelemburg gait: Observed in patients with coxarthrosis or gluteus medius weakness, characterized by a pelvic drop towards the swinging side and a compensatory trunk tilt towards the affected side. In the frontal plane, the contralateral drop during swing phase due to homolateral gluteus medius failure is usually accompanied by a homolateral trunk tilt. This becomes a Trendelenburg gait pattern. Alterations in the pelvis, hip, knee and foot can affect the angle of foot progression, which can result in a loss of proper alignment during gait.

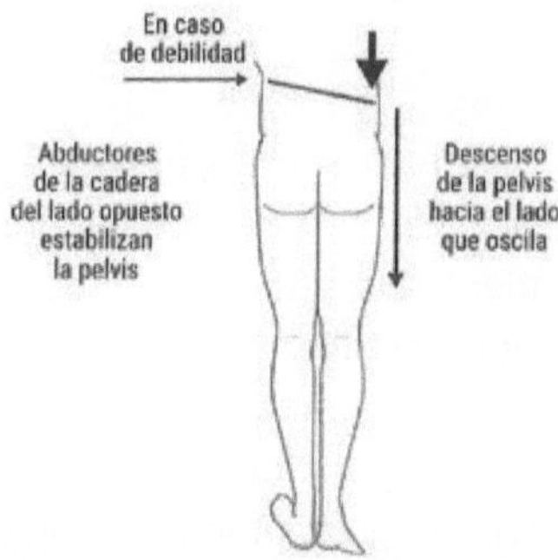

Figure 28. Trandelemburg gait pattern (74).

- Cerebellar ataxic gait (staggering, zigzagging, inebriated):

Ataxic gait is common in people with cerebellar damage. Cerebellar dysfunction can have a variety of causes, such as vascular problems, trauma, infection, toxicity, metabolic, immune or tumor disorders. People with cerebellar ataxia show an unsteady gait with irregular steps and a wide base of support (feet too far apart for balance). They cannot walk in a straight line and have an irregular gait. They walk with legs apart and arms away from the body, with short, unsteady steps, as if they were drunk, and tend to fall backwards, but do not have Romberg's sign. The trunk sways to both sides and they tend to deviate to one side when walking. Depending on the location of the cerebellar lesions, clinical symptoms vary:

- Lesions in the vermis, flocculonodular lobe or fastigial nucleus mainly affect balance and gait (staggering, zigzagging).
- Hemispheric lesions are characterized by limb dysmetry without a clear imbalance of the body axis.

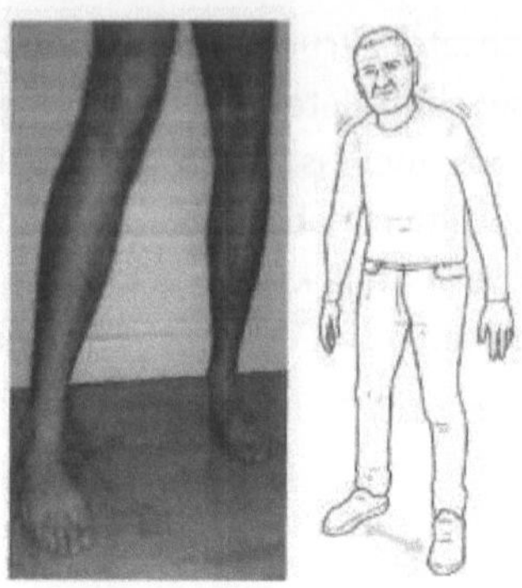

Figure 29. Ataxic gait pattern (74).

- Ataxic tabetic gait (heel strike): Due to proprioceptive sensitivity disorders, the patient raises the limbs too much and drops them abruptly, producing heel strike.
- Apraxic gait: Apraxic gait is a type of movement disorder that has several distinctive features. One of the main difficulties faced by people with this type of gait is the initiation of movement. Patients often have trouble taking the first step, which can cause them to stand still for several seconds before they are able to start walking. Another notable feature is the slowing of walking speed. Unlike a normal gait, people with apraxic gait move at a much slower pace. Their steps tend to be short and uncoordinated, which prevents them from maintaining a steady, flowing pace. Shuffling is another common feature of apraxic gait. Patients do not lift their feet off the ground properly when walking, which causes their feet to drag. This shuffling can increase the risk of trips and falls, as the feet can easily catch on obstacles on the ground. To compensate for instability, people with an apraxic gait often increase their base of support. This means that they walk with their feet wider apart than normal, which helps them maintain balance. However, this adaptation can make the gait appear more awkward and uncoordinated. In addition, people with an apraxic gait face great difficulty when making turns. Changing direction can be especially challenging, as the coordination required to execute these movements is often impaired. This difficulty is compounded by loss of postural control of the trunk, causing the trunk to lean or sway inappropriately when walking.

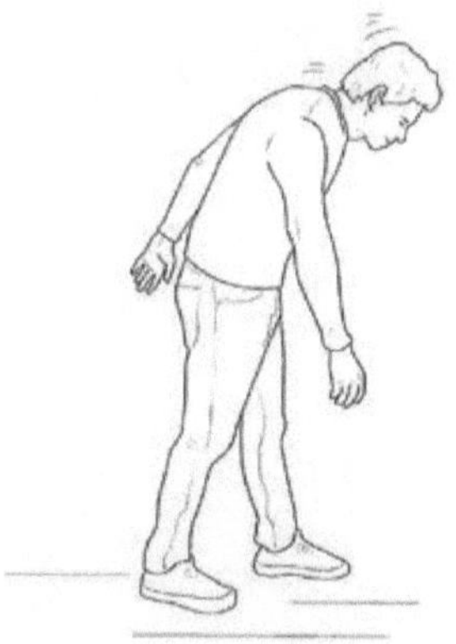

Figure 30. Apraxic gait (74).

- Dancing gait: Characteristic of multiple sclerosis, it combines stiffness and lack of coordination with spastic and ataxic movements.
- Spastic or scissors gait: It is observed in bilateral lesions of the pyramidal pathway. In these cases, the legs are slightly flexed at the knees and move with a notable adduction of the muscles due to the great hypertonicity of the adductors. The patient walks with short strides and knees together, which causes the lower limbs to tend to cross during gait (hence also called "scissors gait"). The trunk is constantly swaying laterally in order to move forward. The movement of the limbs is slow and rigid, which implies a high risk of falling. Movement is performed with great difficulty and effort, which involves considerable energy expenditure and early fatigue. Since gait impairment is one of the symptoms that most impairs the quality of life of people with brain injury, it is necessary to objectively identify the altered motor patterns during gait in order to restore them and thus improve the symmetry of the locomotor pattern and the independence of patients.

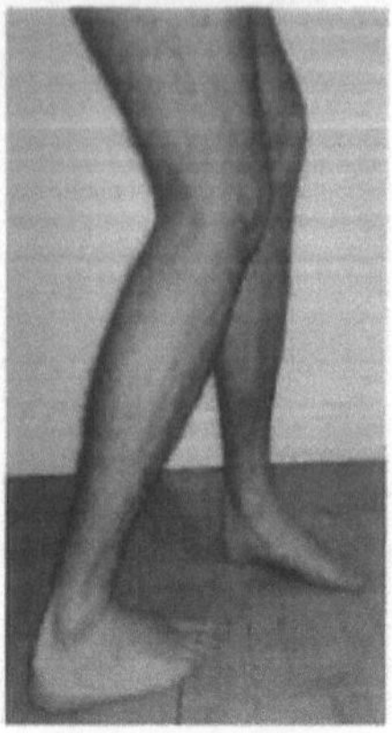

Figure 31. Spastic or scissors gait pattern (74).

- Cockerel gait: It is characterized by support on the toes and oscillation of the lower limb with rotation and inclination movements of the trunk.
- Antalgic gait: Due to pain, the stance phase is shortened and the oscillation of the contralateral limb is reduced.
- Chalan gait: Type of antalgic gait in which the limb is gently supported on the ground to avoid heel strike, typical in sciatica.
- Metatarsal gait: Avoid forefoot support due to forefoot pain.
- Star gait: In vestibular disorders, patients tend to deviate towards the affected side during gait.
- Mallard gait (duck, comedy king, penguin): Observed in muscular dystrophies and myopathic syndromes. Muscular dystrophies and myopathic syndromes are caused by genetic disorders leading to muscle dysfunction and progressive weakness, evidenced by dystrophic changes on muscle biopsy. These conditions are due to mutations affecting genes of the dystrophin-glycoprotein complex (encompassing the sarcolemma) or genes involved in α-dystroglycan glycosylation, RNA splicing and other enzymatic activities.

  Duchenne muscular dystrophy is one of the most common and severe types of muscular dystrophy. The muscle weakness in this disease primarily affects the trunk and pelvic girdle, significantly impacting the gluteal musculature. This pattern of weakness produces a characteristic gait known as "waddling gait".

  - Characteristics of Duchenne gait:

- Trunk sway: Patients show significant trunk sway when walking due to weakness of the gluteal muscles.
- Separation of the feet: To compensate for weakness and maintain stability, patients walk with their feet apart.
- Lumbar hyperlordosis: Weakness of the trunk musculature causes excessive curvature of the lower back.

• Gowers' sign: When asking the patient to sit up from a sitting position or from the floor, it is typical to observe Gowers' sign. This sign consists of the patient using his hands to "climb" up his own legs, leaning on his knees in order to stand up due to muscle weakness in the pelvic girdle and trunk.

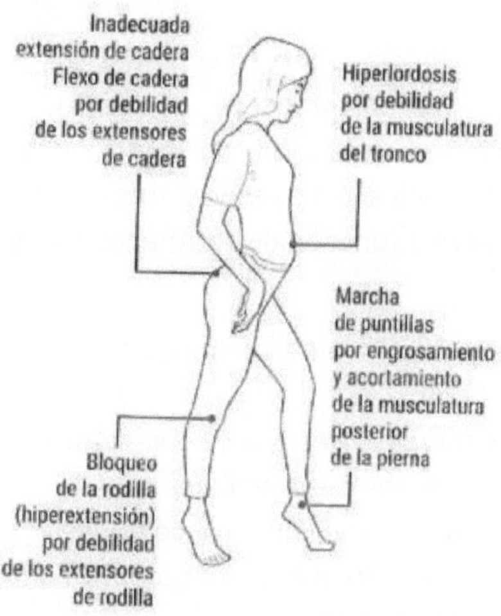

Figure 32. Duck or mallard gait pattern (74).

- Salutatory (saluting) gait: Seen in patients with hip flexion or quadriceps palsy, compensated with plantar flexors of the foot and trunk movements.
- Extensor jerk gait (gluteus maximus palsy): The patient pushes the trunk backward after initial contact to maintain hip extension.
- Hysterical gait: changing and with mixed characteristics, without correlation with physical findings, indicates a psychogenic disorder.
- Charlot's (clown's) gait: Due to excessive femoral external rotation, the patient walks with the toes pointing outward.
- Choreic gait: Broad, continuous movements of the face, trunk and limbs, as in Sydenham's chorea and Huntington's disease.

- Dystonic gait: In dystonia, with support on the external edge of the foot, excessive plantar flexion, or excessive elevation of the lower limbs. In advanced stages, they may present torsion of the trunk and increased lumbar lordosis.

11.5. Gait training

Gait training after an injury or bodily dysfunction must be carried out in a progressive and individualized manner. This type of training aims to restore the ability to walk efficiently and safely, which is essential for the autonomy and quality of life of the affected person. The essential aspects to be taken into account during this process are described below (82).

The ability to ambulate is essential for interaction with the environment and the maintenance of health. Various pathological processes can alter or reduce the ability to locomote, so the primary objective of rehabilitation is to recover this ability in the best possible condition. To achieve a functional gait, the following requirements must be met (82):

- Weight bearing: The lower extremities must be able to support the weight of the body.
- Locomotor rhythm: It is necessary to generate a walking rhythm that propels the body in the desired direction.
- Dynamic balance: Maintaining balance during movement is crucial.
- Adaptation to the environment: The gait must adapt to environmental demands and task changes.

Gait training should be based on a prior systematic evaluation that identifies functional alterations and their possible causes. This allows the design of physiotherapeutic interventions aimed at correcting specific deviations. Due to the diversity of patients and conditions, strategies can vary widely (82).

- Progressive gait training: Progressive training focuses on developing an upright posture and is based on a progression scheme that gradually increases in difficulty. Initially, broad bases of support and a low center of gravity are used. Subsequently, the base of support is reduced and the center of gravity is raised to increase the challenge.

- Mobility: Initially, movement is manually assisted until a certain position is reached.
- Stability: We work on maintaining the posture against gravity.
- Dynamic Stability: Focuses on maintaining balance while shifting weight during movements.
- Ability: The aim is to reach the posture with good motor control and stability.
- Training progresses from guided or assisted movements to active, then resisted and independent movements. The progression and selection of exercises must be individualized.

The following aspects should be worked on (82):

- Pelvic Lift
  - Initial Position: The patient lies supine with hips and knees flexed and feet resting on a mat.
  - Execution: Lifting the pelvis from this position strengthens the gluteal and lumbar extensor musculature, and aids in the transfer from seated to standing.
  - Progression: Begin with the arms in abduction to increase the base of support and manual assistance. Then, move to active exercises with resistance applied on the iliac crests or knees.
- Quadrupedia
  - Starting Position: Support on knees and palms of hands, with elbows extended.
  - Execution: This posture allows weight bearing on the hands and the lower portion of the trunk. It can be progressed by performing mediolateral and craniocaudal displacements of the trunk, and elevations of the limbs.
- Sitting
  - Initial Position: Static and dynamic postural control with hips and knees in flexion and feet resting on a surface.
  - Execution: Progress from a supine position to a seated position with hand support. Then, perform body weight shifts in various directions with less arm support.
- Bipedestación

- Initial Position: The patient should be adapted to an upright posture, starting with exercises in a standing position and performing body weight shifts in different directions.
- Execution: Progressing with steps forward or backward and climbing steps. Incorporate balance activities and adjust postures to improve stability and motor control.

- Seated to standing transfer
    - Execution: Involves moving the trunk forward with the feet slightly behind the knees. The therapist may manually assist the patient to facilitate the movement.
- Repetitive training and partial body weight support: A common modality is repetitive training with partial body weight support, which can be performed with a rolling walkway or robotic devices. In both cases, the patient's weight is partially suspended while walking, allowing the therapist to assist with altered movements and provide stability.
- Training should focus on specific gait functions:
    - Weight Reception: Work on hip extension, pelvic descent, knee flexion and ankle plantar flexion.
    - Propulsion and Advancement: Focused on hip extension, knee flexion, controlled foot drop and plantar flexion to facilitate lower extremity swing.
    - Stability and Alignment: Ensures alignment of the center of gravity with the joints and controls ground reaction forces to maintain stability during gait.

Gait training is a complex process that must be tailored to the individual patient's needs. Accurate assessment, appropriate exercise progression and attention to specific gait functions are essential to achieve effective rehabilitation and improve patients' quality of life.

12. Bibliographic References

1. Gallego, T. (2007). Theoretical bases and fundamentals of physical therapy. Panamericana. ISBN: 978-84-7903-976-9
2. Meliá, J.F. (2008). History of physiotherapy. ISBN: 978-84-612-2984-0
3. Raposo, I., et al. (2001). Physiotherapy in Spain during the nineteenth and twentieth centuries until the integration into university schools of physiotherapy. 23(4): 206-217.
4. Chillón, R., Rebollo, J., Meroño, A.J. (2008). Approach to the history of Spanish physiotherapy from documentary sources. Revista cuestiones de fisioterapia. 37(3).
5. Ministry of Health and Consumption (2002). Real decreto 1001/2002, de 27 de septiembre, por el que se aprueban los estatutos generales del consejo general de colegios de fisioterapeutas. Madrid.
6. Bispo, J.P. (2021). Physiotherapy in health systems: theoretical framework and foundations for an integral practice. Collective Health Journal. ISSN: 1669-2381
7. Vargas, M.D. (2020). Clinical history and assessment in physical therapy. NPunto Journal. 31(3).
8. Daza, J. (2007). Clinical-functional evaluation of human body movement. Panamericana. ISBN: 958-9181-61-4
9. Vicente, M.T., et al. (2018). Pain assessment: comparative review of scales and questionnaires. Journal of the Spanish Pain Society. 24(4): 228-236
10. Chaitow L. (2001). Manual therapy: Assessment and diagnosis. Madrid: McGraw-Hill Interamericana. ISBN: 9788448603595
11. Borrel, F. (2017). Clinical interviewing: Manual of practical strategies. SemFYC. ISBN: 84-96216-44-6
12. Karcioglu, O., et al. (2018). A systematic review of the pain scales in adults: Which to use?. American Journal of Emergency Medicine.
13. Petty, N., Moore, A. (2003). Neuromusculoskeletal exploration and assessment: A handbook for therapists. McGraw-Hill. ISBN: 84-486-0560-8
14. Bickley, L., Szilagyi, P. (2017). Guide to physical examination and medical history 12th edition. Wolters Kluwer. ISBN: 978-84-16781-67-6.

15.Herrero, V., Delgado, S., Bandrés, F., Ramírez, M.V., Capdevila, L. (2018). Pain assessment. Comparative review of scales and questionnaires. Revista sociedad española del dolor. 25(4): 228-236.
16.Viel, E. (2006). Physiotherapeutic diagnosis. Conception and application in free and hospital practice. Barcelona Masson. ISBN: 9788445807750.
17.Santamaría, A., García, E., Pérez, M., Pacheco, C. (2020). Physiotherapeutic diagnosis based on the General theory of systems. FisioGía. 7(1): 11-17.
18.Jiménez, E. (2016). Methodological guide to elaborate the physiotherapeutic diagnosis according to the International Classification of Functioning (ICF), disability and health. Gaceta médica Bolivia. 39(1): 46-52.
19.Jiménez, M.T., González, P., Martín, J.M. (2002). The international classification of disability and health functioning. Revista española publica. 76(4): 271-279.
20.Vázquez, J.L. (2001). International classification of functioning, disability and health (WHO). Ministry of labor and social affairs. ISBN 9241545445
21.World Health Organization (WHO) (2001). The International Classification Functioning, Disability and Health. ISBN 9241545429
22.Díaz, M.J. (2005). The equivalence of assessment tests with the international classification of functionality, disability and health. Revista iberoamericana fisioterapia kinesiología. 8(1):36-43.
23.Trigás, M., Ferreira, L., Meijide, H. (2011). Functional assessment scales in the elderly. Galicia clinica. 72(1):11-16.
24.Bernejo, F., Porta, J., Díaz, J., Martínez, P. (2008). More than one hundred scales in neurology. 2nd edition Madrid: Series Manuales.
25.Mathoney, F.I., Barthel D.W. (1965). Functional evaluation: The Barthel Index: a simple index of independence useful in scoring improvement in the rehabilitation of the chronically ill. Maryland state medical journal; 1965.
26.Lawton, M.P., Brody, E.M. (1970). Assessment or folder people: self-maintaining and instrumental activities of daily living. Nursing Research. 19(3): 278.
27.Cabañero, M.J. Cabrero, J., Richart, M., Muñoz, C. (2008). Structured review of activities of daily living measures in older people. Journal of Geriatrics and Gerontology. 43(5): 271-83.

28.Linn, M.W., Linn, B.S. The rapid disability rating scale 2. Journal of the American geriatrics society, 1982; 30: 378-382.
29.Teng, E., Becker, B.W., Woo, E., Knopman, D.S., Cummings, J.L., Lu, P.H. (2010). Utility of the functional activities questionnaire for distinguishing mild cognitive impairment from very mild Alzheimer's disease. Alzheimer Dis Assoc Disord. 24(4): 348-53.
30.Jiménez, P.E., López, F., Portilla, J.C., Pedrera, M.A., Lavado, J.M., et al. (2012). Assessment of instrumental activities of daily living after stroke using the Lawton and Brody scale. Neurological Journal. 55(6): 337-42.
31.Gutiérrez, E.T., Meneses, A.L., Bermúdez, P.A., Gutiérrez, A., Padilla, A. (2022). Usefulness of the Dowton and Tinetti scales in the classification of fall risk in older adults in primary health care. Downtown medical act. 16(1).
32.Forner, I., Muñoz, J., Forner, A., Gisbert Grifo, M., Delgado, M. (2004). Valuation of body damage in spinal cord injury: differences between quadriplegics and paraplegics. Rehabilitación Integral. 38(2):51-58.
33.Paolinelli, G., González, P., Doniez, E., Donoso, T., Salinas, V. (2001) Functional assessment instrument for disability in rehabilitation: Reliability study and clinical experience with the use of the Functional Independence Measure. Medical Journal Chile. 129(1): 23-31.
34.Mirallas, J.A., Real, M.C. (2003). Barthel Index or Functional Independence Measure? Rehabilitation. 37(3):152-7.
35.Vilagut, G., Ferrer, M., Rajmil, Rebollo, P., Permanyer, P., Quintana, J.M., et al. (2005). The Spanish SF-36 Health Questionnaire: a decade of experience and new developments. Gaceta Sanit. 19(2): 135-150.
36.O'Connor, M., Davitt, J.K. (2012). The Outcome and Assessment Information Set (OASIS): a review of validity and reliability. Home Health Care Serv Q. 31(4):267-301.
37.López, A., Lacida, M., Rodríguez, S. (2004), Cuestionarios, test e índices para la valoración del paciente. Andalusian Health Service.
38.Feldman, A.B., Haley, S.M., Coryell, J. (1990). Concurrent adn construct validity of the pediatric evaluation of disability inventory. Phys Ther. 70(10):602-10.
39.Reuben, D.B., Siu, A.L., Kimpau, S. (1992) The Predictive Validity of Self-Report and Performance-based Measures of Function and Health. J Gerontol. 47(4): M106-10.

40.Nagi, S.Z. (1976). An epidemiology of disability among adults in the United States. Milbank Mem Fund Q Health Soc. 54(4): 439-67.
41.Ortega, M.A., Herce, M.B., Valiñas, F., Mariscal, N., López, M.A., Cubo, E. (2013). Study of the impact of rural or urban environment on residual disability after stroke. Clinical Nursing. 23(5):182-8. 92.
42.López, F., Jiménez, M.A., Luengo, E., Blanco, A., Márquez, J., Bravo, S et al. (2011). Descriptive study of patients attended in a stroke unit in the Community of Extremadura. Enfermería Intensiva. 22(4): 138-43.
43.Schuling, J., De Haan, R., Limburg, M., Groenier, K.H. (1993). The Frenchay Activities In-dex. Assessment of functional status in stroke patients. Stroke. 24(8):1173-7.
44.Hobart, J., Lamping, D., Fitzpatrick, R., Riazi, A., Thompson, A. (2001). The Multiple Sclerosis Impact Scale (MSIS-29) A new patient-based outcome measure. Brain. 124(5):962-73.
45.Bushnik, T. (2011). Expanded Disability Status Scale. Encyclopedia of Clinical Neuropsychology. Springer New York. 997-9.
46.Campos, T.S., Rodríguez, F., Esteban, J., Vázquez, P.C., Mora, J.S., Carmona, A.C. (2010). Spanish adaptation of the revised Amyotrophic Lateral Sclerosis Functional Rating Scale (ALSFRS-R). Amyotroph Lateral Scler. 11(5):475-7.
47.Boer, A.G., Wijker, W., Speelman, J.D., De Haes, J.C. (1996). Quality of life in patients with Parkinson's disease: development of a questionnaire. Journal of Neurology, Neurosurgery & Psychiatry. 61(1):70-4.
48.Buendía, A., Mazuecos, J., Camacho, J.M. (2018). Anatomy and physiology of the skin. Manual of dermatology 2nd ed. (1): 2-27. ISBN: 978-84-7885-628-2.
49.Zarco, A., Torres, M., Peña, S., López, M.A. (2024). Manual for the exploration of the skin and its annexes. UNAM, FES Zaragoza.
50.Lapunzina, P., Aiello, H. (2002). Manual of normal and pathological anthropometry. Editorial Masson. ISBN: 84-458-1122-3.
51.Sandoval, M.C., Camargo, D.M., Galván, D.M., Hernández, N.O., García, L.J. (2004). Evaluation of volumetric and perimetric methods. Salud UIS. 36(1).
52.Esparza, F., Vaquero, R. (2023). Anthropometry: Fundamentals for application and interpretation. Mc Graw Hill. ISBN: 9788419544896.
53.Garlito, H., Galán, M., Manzarbeitia, P., Cabello, J. (2024). Flatfoot and other foot disorders. Pediatría integral. 28(2): 241-247.

54.Palazzi, S. (1972). Exploration and assessment of nerve injuries of the hand. Catalan society of orthopedic surgery and traumatology. 820-821.
55.Echeverría, M. (2006). Validation of a new method for digital surface analysis. Cir. plást. iberolatinoam. 32(2): 71-82.
56.Cardoso, M.A., Moreira, O., Silva, A., Quintanilha, G., Sacristan, L., Paiva, F. (2010). Profile of neuropathic pain. Brazilian Journal of Anesthesiology. 60(2).
57.Rohen, J.W., Yokochi, C., Lutjen, E. (2021). Atlas of human anatomy: Photographic study of the human body. 9th Edition Elsevier. ISBN: 978-84-1382-033-0
58.Angulo, M.T., Dobao, C. (2010). Clinical biomechanics: joint biomechanics. Reduca (Nursing, physiotherapy and podiatry). 2(3): 14-31. ISSN: 1989-5305.
59.Donald, A. (2022). Kinesiology of the musculoskeletal system: fundamentals for rehabilitation 3rd edition. Panamericana. ISBN: 978-8829932788.
60.Arvelo, N.(2012). Articular kinematics. Journal of the Venezuelan society of morphological sciences. 18(1).
61.Granero, J. (2010). Manual of physical examination of the locomotor system. Medical and marketing communications. ISBN: 978-84-693-8580-7.
62.Ricard, F., Sallé, J. (2007). Treatise on Osteopathy. Editorial Panamericana 3rd Edition. ISBN: 9788479036935
63.López, C. (2022). Neurodynamics in Clinical Practice. 2nd edition. Ed. Wolters Kluwer. ISBN 9788418892066.
64.Vega, J. (1999). Joint and muscle proprioceptors. Biomechanics. 7(13): 79-93.
65.Kapandji, A.I. (2006). Articular physiology volume 1: Upper limb. Editorial Panamericana 6th Edition. ISBN: 9788498350029.
66.Kapandji, A.I. (2012). Fisiología articular tomo 3: Tronco y raquis. Editorial Panamericana 6th Edition. ISBN: 9788498354607.
67.Dufour, M. (2008). Physical examination and joint assessment. Kinesiotherapy-Physical Medicine. 29(1): 1-23.
68.Kaltenborn, F.M. (2001). Manual therapy extremities. McGraw-Hill Publishers. ISBN: 9788448603359
69.Maigne, R.(2005).spine and extremities manipulations. Editorial Norma. ISBN: 84-8451-021-2.

70.Sala, M., Gómez, J.J., Cazorla, J. (2019). Assessment in physiotherapy. Editorial Bradu. ISBN: 978-84-18005-01-5.
71.Palmer, M., Epler, M. (2002). Fundamentals of musculoskeletal assessment techniques. Editorial Paidotribo. ISBN: 84-8019-657-2.
72.Sánchez, J.J. (2005). Biomechanics of normal and pathological human gait. Instituto de biomecánica valencia. ISBN: 9788495448125.
73.Cerda, L. (2010). Evaluation of the patient with gait disorder. Revista hospital clínico universitario chine. 21: 326-36.
74.Molina, F., Carratalá, M. (2020). Human gait: Biomechanics, evaluation and pathology. Editorial panamericana. ISBN: 9788491104056.
75.Lord, S., Halligan, P., Wade, D. (1998). Visual gait analysis: the development of a clinical assessment and scale. Clinical Rehabilitation. 12(2): 107-119.
76.Murciano, M., Periñán, M.J., Corral, I., Alamo, V., Ferrand, P., Barrera, J.M. (2022). Development of the Spanish version of the Wisconsin Gait Scale. Consistency analysis of temporo-spatial parameters with gait assessment in stroke patients. Elsevier. 56(2): 133-141.
77.Daly, J., Nethery, J., McCabe, J., Brenner, I., Rogers, J., Gansen, J., et al. (2009). Development and testing of the Gait Assessment and Intervention Tool (G.A.I.T.): a measure of coordinated gait components. J Neurosci Methods. 15;178(2):334-9.
78.Tinetti, M.E., Williams, T., Mayewski, R. (1986). "Fall risk index for elderly patients based on number of chronic disabilities". American Journal of Medicine 80 (3): 429-434.
79.Vanswearingen, J., Paschal, K., Bonino, P., Yang, J.F. (1996). The Modified Gait Abnormality Rating Scale for Recognizing the Risk of Recurrent Falls in Community-Dwelling Elderly Adults. Physical Therapy. 76(9):994-1002.
80.Chaler, J., Garreta, R., Muller, B. (2005). Instrumental techniques of diagnosis and assessment in rehabilitation: Study of walking. Rehabilitation. 39(6): 305-314.
81.Martí, I., García, R., Gorría, N., Aguilera, S. (2022). Gait disorders. Protocolos asociación española de pediatría. 1:218-293.
82.Cerda, L. (2014). Management of gait disorder in the older adult. Clinical medical journal condes. 25(2): 265-275.

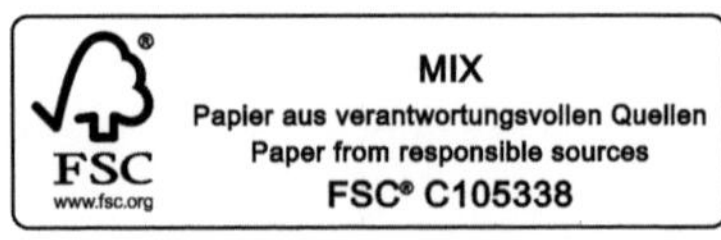

Printed by Books on Demand GmbH, Norderstedt / Germany